Invisibly Allergic

Invisibly Allergic

A Memoir
of
Survival, Advocacy, and Change

By Zoë Slaughter

First Edition, Copyright © 2025 by Zoë Slaughter

Design by Caitlin Nunavath

Edited by Julia Nusbaum

All rights reserved. No part of this book may be reproduced or transmitted in any form or by any means, electronic or mechanical, including photocopying, recording, or by any information storage and retrieval system, without prior written permission from the publisher, except in the case of brief quotations used in reviews or articles.

ISBN 979-8-9937151-1-7

Published by Invisibly Allergic

Louisville, Kentucky

www.invisiblyallergic.com

CONTENTS

Introduction / *1*

1: Preschool Years / *13*

2: Middle & High School Years / *36*

3: College and Early 20s / *48*

4: Anaphylaxis at the Allergist / *67*

5: Life After Anaphylaxis: Finding Humor and Healing / *91*

6: Decoding Food Labels / *110*

7: Navigating Cross-Contact / *135*

8: Accommodations / *165*

9: Non-Food Products / *191*

10: Media's Impact on Food Allergy Awareness / *210*

11: The Intersection of Mental Health and Food Allergies / *231*

12: The Future of Allergy Care / *297*

A Final Word / *311*

Acknowledgements / *316*

INTRODUCTION

My introduction to food allergies began in early childhood with my own peanut allergy. It evolved through adolescence and into adulthood, and with hindsight I can see how profoundly my identity has been shaped by my food allergy. Along with this personal evolution, societal attitudes and shifting medical advancements have also played a significant role in molding my perspective on living with food allergies.

Over the years, I've observed a remarkable shift in how food allergies are understood and managed, compared to just a decade ago. This progress leaves me optimistic about the future as food allergy research and awareness continue to grow from their still-developing foundations. It's only recently, in my thirties, that I've started to recognize how my food allergy may have quietly shaped my sense of self, often limiting me in ways I hadn't realized.

At the same time, recent years have brought more empowerment to the food allergy community as a whole. We're advocating for greater inclusion, stronger regulations, and improved practices, while also addressing gaps in education, policy, mental health resources, and self-advocacy tools. Food allergies and chronic conditions affect the entire family, making support groups and community connections an essential resource for both patients and caregivers.

Like much medical care in the US, access to resources regarding food allergies is far from equitable. Systemic inequalities impact the food allergy space, leaving low-income and marginalized families without access to the care, life-saving medications, or comprehensive allergy education they deserve. Research continues to highlight how these communities are disproportionately affected, experiencing higher rates of food allergies and related complications.

I embarked on this writing journey because my food allergy knowledge, both innate and acquired, felt too big to share in everyday exchanges. A book was the only way I felt I could give it shape and clarity. Through writing this memoir, I've realized that there are people who genuinely care and want to understand the food allergy experience, including mine. Recognizing that has been deeply therapeutic.

I hope this book helps readers to better navigate their own food allergy journeys or to support loved ones in managing food allergies, intolerances, celiac disease, or any allergic condition. Anyone can develop a food allergy at any time, and it's long overdue that we treat these realities with the seriousness they deserve.

In these pages, you'll find my own personal stories woven with statistics and other people's powerful narratives to paint a holistic picture, with some names changed for privacy. There's a psychological toll that comes with managing a life-threatening condition—particularly one that isn't often visible, which is how I began my food allergy blogging journey back in 2017 and why I titled it *Invisibly Allergic*.

To help you navigate this journey, each chapter includes closing thoughts, often with additional information and action items that build on the stories and insights shared. This way, the personal anecdotes, facts, and resources lay the foundation, and the prompts and reflections help you deepen your personal awareness.

Here, you'll encounter the heaviness of discussing death by anaphylaxis alongside lighter moments where I use humor to gently soften the edges of my valid fears. In short, these pages reflect the full spectrum of one person's food allergy experiences.

My hope is that these pages will allow others, who so rarely feel seen, to feel seen, because I know that as I searched for this feeling of relatability in extended personal narratives, I came up short. For a long time, I never considered that sharing so much of my allergy experience was even possible—until I met others like me and realized, *wow, there's a real need for this kind of openness and insight.* It's important for everyone—food allergic or not—to better understand life with food allergies in a way that resonates.

I know many of my friends and family want to learn more, as do the broader circles of others with allergies. However, since the responsibility often falls on the allergic person to convey their experience in a way that's both digestible and builds understanding, it can be difficult to do so without depleting our energy. Advocacy is a daily necessity for us in many ways, and as many of us have likely experienced, it's something we deeply want to share, but it can also be equally exhausting, dark, and emotionally draining.

While conveying information about our specific food allergies can help others better understand the condition, it's important to emphasize that the way individuals manage their allergies and experience reactions varies enormously. This can be difficult to grasp, even within the allergy community itself. For example, one person's definition of being "very careful" when managing their allergies might look completely different from another's. Some individuals may feel comfortable being around their food allergens in their homes, and with family, and friends eating them nearby, while others may need to avoid spaces with their allergens entirely.

These inconsistencies in practice can lead to confusion, which often diminishes the gravity of life-threatening conditions and can make people feel too confused to attempt to accommodate. It's important to remember that everyone's allergies are different, and that's the key takeaway. Terms like "cautious" or "severe" are often used to describe allergies, but they are frequently misapplied or left unexplained.

For instance, someone might describe their food intolerance as "deadly" to get the point across, when in reality what they're experiencing is intensely painful gastrointestinal distress. While this can be horrible, completely disrupt their day, and deserves care, it is not the same as potentially fatal anaphylaxis, an allergic reaction in which the immune system overreacts to a harmless substance, and should not be described that way.

Similarly, conditions like celiac disease are sometimes referred to as "an allergy" or "gluten allergy" to be taken seriously, especially in restaurant settings. You technically can't have a "gluten allergy" in the same way you can have a wheat allergy that causes an IgE-mediated anaphylactic reaction, but people sometimes use the phrase because it communicates quickly that their body cannot safely tolerate gluten. Accidental gluten ingestion in celiac disease can cause long-term bodily harm. Only a true anaphylactic reaction, such as from a wheat allergy, requires immediate epinephrine intervention.

Whether intentionally or not, our language matters because misusing terms like "deadly" can dilute their meaning and confuse allergic response protocols for those with truly life-threatening conditions. An *everybody* problem can quickly become a *nobody* problem, when in reality, we can speak honestly about the reality of these reactions and deserve to be taken seriously regardless.

My goal is to better convey the allergy experience in a way that's easier to understand and clearer. These nuances in language are exactly why I've chosen to focus on sharing my specific experiences in this book, rather than relying on subjective labels or expecting readers to read between the lines.

As much as I wish everything here could be ever-relevant, this book serves as a time capsule. While much of the factual data and protocols I share will inevitably become outdated in some way, this text will forever offer an important foundational base of knowledge that can be added onto. The field of food allergies is constantly shifting, with new research and regulations reshaping our understanding and medical practices. With that said, I want to include a disclaimer encouraging everyone to verify the statistics and advancements I mention throughout, as I am not a medical professional and medical advice and therapeutics will undoubtedly shift over time.

Such as, many in the medical field are now advising that, in certain circumstances, going to the ER after using epinephrine may not always be necessary. For years, the protocol was sound—if you use epinephrine, you must go to the hospital or urgent care immediately. This adjustment illustrates an important point: there is no across-the-board approach to managing food allergies.

Guidelines and best practices can shift from year to year as our understanding deepens. What works or is recommended one year may change the next—making it essential to stay informed and flexible. The nature of food allergies is complex and highly individual—no two people's experiences are exactly the same, nor are they guaranteed to remain the same over time. What follows in these chapters is not a definitive guide, but an exploration of the many facets of living with food allergies.

Whether you're a parent navigating the challenges of raising a child with allergies, an educator fostering inclusivity, a food industry professional seeking to improve, an ally wondering how to support, or simply someone who enjoys reading memoirs and nonfiction, this book is for you. It's also for the food allergy individuals out there—whether you're newly diagnosed or have lived with allergies since childhood. You're not alone, and many people want to see us live full, vibrant lives.

To the readers managing multiple food allergies, I want to acknowledge the complexity and vigilance your daily life requires. To those with one allergen, like me, I hope this book also reflects the hyperawareness we feel, knowing how quickly circumstances can change due to the looming threat of anaphylaxis.

To those in the thick of managing food trauma or intense anxiety around food allergies, I'm here to reassure you: it's okay to take things one step at a time. Mastering food allergy management tools won't happen overnight. Your support systems, education, and adaptability will carry you through at your own pace. I've returned to the same resources multiple times because I knew I couldn't absorb it all at once. If that sounds familiar, I encourage you to treat this book the same way. You don't have to read it once and move on. Highlight pages, underline, take notes, or use whatever method helps you.

The truth is, living with food allergies can be isolating, and there's a constant lack of control we must learn to accept. Allergies can make us feel small, like a boat in a narrow canal, navigating spaces not made for our shape. But they can also be a source of immense connection, empathy, and adaptability, among many other strengths. I've realized that problem-solving, creativity, and thinking outside the box are skills I've cultivated out of necessity due to my allergy, and they've become unexpected gifts I can carry into all parts of life, whether or not allergies are at the center. Community is essential for everyone; it is a form of medicine. We heal from one another in connection, not operating in isolation.

As a peanut-allergic adult who is cross-contact allergic to trace amounts, airborne, and has a food allergy disability, my condition impacts all aspects of my life. I've identified as having a food allergy disability for many years now, yet I still tear up when I use the term *food allergy disability* to explain myself because it feels so accurate.

To me, it encompasses the experience I've lived with for 35+ years. Yet, until recently, I never had the phrase to describe it. When I stumbled upon this terminology, I felt whole. No one ever told me I had a food allergy disability. I had to claim that for myself. I spent years waiting for validation that never came. And that sense of invisibility, of hovering in a gray area, is something I know many people can relate to. Gray is hard. It's uncomfortable sometimes. Life doesn't always hand us neat categories or clear paths, so sometimes we have to squeeze our way through, forging something that feels truer to us.

I now have a community where I can fully embrace my food allergy journey without needing to over-explain or shrink myself. And that's a wonderful feeling. I'm not saying everything is easy—depression, anxiety, and panic attacks still show up, shaped in part by the weight of my allergy and other autoimmune conditions. But all of it is real. All of it matters. And all of it belongs in the story.

I'm so proud to be where I am today. I've spent more than five years working on this book, and I'm finally able to call it "done enough" to get it out into the world. I tend to explain my allergy in flexible terms because I don't know what my allergy will be like in 5, 10, or 20 years. Maybe it'll be the same, maybe I'll use a new form of treatment and get additional food freedom to some extent, who knows? And that's okay. I don't need permanence.

A reality for the food allergy community is that one misstep—whether it's a mislabeling on a food package or an error made by someone else—can quickly lead to a life-threatening situation. Death is always a potential outcome, and things can change for us in an instant. It's the hand we've been dealt, just as with any other life-threatening condition.

I've witnessed how the food allergy community comes together in the wake of every tragedy, feeling the loss deeply as if it were personal. Because it could happen to any of us, the grief feels familial. At its core, there's a helplessness that binds us together, creating a connection even when we don't know the person affected. We've all faced moments of fear, and it's this shared vulnerability that unites us, reminding us of our fragility.

What's become clear to me over the years is that communication around food allergies evolves over time—and varies depending on age, stage of life, and relationship dynamics. Toddlers, for example, are often impulsive and might grab food off someone's plate or off the floor without realizing it could be harmful to them. In those cases, managing allergies requires a vigilant adult's oversight and age-appropriate boundaries, rather than complex explanations.

As kids grow into tweens and teens, the conversation shifts again. Now they're managing allergies in peer environments, making independent choices at school, camp, or sleepovers. They may feel pressure to fit in or downplay their needs, ignoring the protocols parents would prefer they follow. This is when empowerment, value-based motivation, confidence, and compassionate support systems become crucial—helping them advocate for their own safety in ways they're actually comfortable with. Fear-based approaches often backfire, so it's important to meet teens where they are and give them options for how they want to take control in order to stay safe.

By adulthood, many of us have developed our own routines, coping strategies, and rules. But even then, we encounter new scenarios: dating, intimacy, pregnancy, parenting, travel, workplace situations. And the conversation around safety doesn't end—it just changes shape. Take kissing, for example. It can present risks at every life stage: a well-meaning relative kissing a child's cheek after snacking on nuts, teens navigating their first romantic encounters, adults sharing a kiss after dinner. I've personally had to set clear boundaries before kissing someone—I'll ask what they've eaten that day and guide the conversation toward safety. Not everyone thinks to consider whether something like a smoothie from four hours ago could still be lingering. But I do.

As a teenager, I wondered if a kiss could trigger a reaction, and decided it was safer to assume yes. I made up my own rules about how much time needed to pass and how many times my partner needed to brush their teeth before I would feel safe. Back then, it felt isolating. Now, it's become a common allergy conversation, with growing awareness around just how many everyday moments can carry life-threatening risk. That visibility matters. We're building something better by naming these situations out loud.

There's science behind it too. A 2006 *Journal of Allergy and Clinical Immunology* paper documented peanut allergen exposure through saliva and showed that brushing teeth, chewing gum, or waiting a few hours can help reduce the allergen, but may not eliminate it completely. The safest route? Eating a non-allergen meal afterward. But even then, food consistency (like sticky nut butters), what's stuck in someone's teeth, and individual risk factors all play a role. There's no one-size-fits-all rule. Each allergic person gets to define their own safety thresholds and boundaries, and it's critical to respect both.

That extends beyond kissing. Risk can come from shared sponges, used towels, a dog's tongue, sharing vape pens, cigarettes or drinks, or touching skin that was recently exposed to an allergen. It may seem uncommon, but trace exposure can absolutely be enough to cause reactions for many people. I use caution around terms like "unusual" or "rare" because they can minimize the legitimate risks we face and add to the disbelief or skepticism we're already up against.

When it comes to managing food allergies, clear communication and openness are essential, because many situations require careful, case-by-case consideration. Sometimes, disability accommodations or health needs can seem to conflict—for example, someone with a dog allergy sitting near a person with a service dog, or a service dog eating peanut butter near someone with a peanut allergy. Or on a plane, a diabetic passenger may need their peanut-containing candy bar they brought while sitting near someone with a peanut allergy. These complex scenarios can't always be neatly solved in advance, but honest communication, empathy, and a willingness to listen help create safer, more respectful spaces for everyone involved.

Ultimately, openness, understanding, and respectful dialogue are key to navigating these complicated realities. Community conversations have raised topics like allergies to sperm or the transmission of allergens to babies through breast milk, though the research isn't yet clear or conclusive. Something as simple as beards or hair can matter—food proteins can get trapped, so washing or trimming might be necessary before getting close.

What matters most is that we stay cautious and communicate clearly, especially during intimate moments. If someone isn't willing to talk about my food allergy respectfully, then honestly, that's not someone I want to be kissing or in close contact with anyway. All I can do is stay prepared with epinephrine because as individuals we can't anticipate every possible scenario. Spontaneous moments—sharing a straw, trying a bite of someone's dessert—can be romantic and fun for others, but potentially life-threatening for someone like me. So I've developed "rules" that work for me, and I communicate them clearly.

I had an incident once where my high school boyfriend forgot he'd eaten Tagalongs—those chocolate-covered peanut butter Girl Scout Cookies. He remembered only after I asked him to run through his food for the day. Mistakes happen, even with the best intentions. But the point is to take it seriously, respond with care, and move forward with more understanding.

At the heart of it, this all comes back to communication, respect, and being empowered to define your own boundaries—whether you're a toddler's parent, a teen navigating dating, or an adult.

We're also beginning to talk more honestly about other nuanced and overlooked stages of life, like senior care and assisted living. Right now, food allergies aren't being handled the way they need to be in these environments—especially adult-onset allergies and conditions like alpha-gal syndrome (AGS), an allergy to a sugar molecule found in the meat of most mammals after being bitten by a tick. The lack of protocols, labeling, and basic awareness in care settings poses a real danger.

Communal living as a whole can be especially difficult, since everyone in the household or facility needs to agree and be fully on board with taking the allergy—or multiple allergies—seriously. In fact, our current hospital cafeterias are often off-limits. Many of us have to bring our own food into these spaces because we can't rely on others to keep us safe or to be knowledgeable and properly trained around our allergens. More often than not, they simply aren't.

That same vulnerability makes it even more urgent to pay attention to the systems people fought for, which were meant to protect us. We can't take for granted that progress will hold. Look at Roe v. Wade. Legislative policies can be reversed, undermined, or stripped away entirely. The current government administration has been swiftly cutting FDA funding and entire departments at a time when the agency is already stretched thin, doing what feels like the bare minimum to safeguard people with food allergies.

These cuts include reductions to critical areas like food labeling enforcement, recalls, and basic food safety checks for hazards like E. coli and salmonella. Environmental protections are also being gutted, including laws and policies that prevent contamination of our air, water, and food supply—directly impacting the safety of the products we consume.

These policy reversals aren't happening in isolation; they echo broader efforts to roll back protections across the board, from women's rights and trans rights to dismantling life-saving scientific cancer research and more. We must balance staying alert while caring for ourselves. It's a strategy designed to leave us overwhelmed, helpless, and numb. But knowing this is what their goal is helps us choose another path. Caring for ourselves, finding joy, and reclaiming power amid this is part of the resistance. Social change is a long game, and we need each other, fully present and resourced, for the road ahead.

Writing these pages has unlocked new avenues of self-growth I never thought possible and uncovered personal struggles I didn't previously recognize as pain points within me. Confronting them has allowed me to address and heal in ways I hadn't imagined. I can't express how appreciative I am that you're taking the time to read this, and I hope you get out of it all I've put into it. Thank you for being a food allergy ally. I hope I can be an ally for you. Whatever goals you're striving for and dreams you're chasing, I hope you go after them wholeheartedly. You have every right to pursue what brings you fulfillment and joy, participate in society, you deserve to see those aspirations realized.

1

PRESCHOOL YEARS

The Beginning

"I SMELL PEANUT BUTTER!" I loudly announced, my nose twitching as I sat at my daycare lunch table. I pushed my little body up off the too-large-for-me vinyl chair. My feet dangled just above the ground before they thudded down, and I hopped off with determination. I leaned across the rectangular lunch table, my eyes wide with urgency, seeking everyone's attention. Confidently, I outstretched my index finger toward the kids sitting with their lunchboxes open on the opposite side of the table. Darting my eyes from person to person, I maintained firm eye contact, scrutinizing their expressions. I waited, feeling the tension build. No one said a word.

The kids stared back at me, mouths slightly agape, their sandwiches frozen halfway to their lips, before they slowly resumed chewing. Thinking back, all the kids at my table were around the age of five, so they wouldn't understand what a peanut allergy is, the same way I didn't. Food allergies weren't openly discussed in the 1990s, and most of what I knew about my peanut allergy came from the sensations I experienced in my body. At that age, I didn't know that peanuts were a naturally occurring food that others could eat safely. In my mind, I thought it was poisonous and dangerous to everyone.

I decided to act bravely. At the head of the sprawling table, my finger stayed poised like an unwavering arrow. Deciding to take one more cautious breath in.

Sniff sniff—

Oh, wow, that's strong! The scent was unmistakable. I felt my nose wrinkle, as I froze mid-inhale, retreating just in time to avoid pulling any more of the allergen-laden air into my lungs. I didn't need to sniff anymore to confirm there were peanuts in the room. There was no doubt about it.

I began to back away, burying my nose in the crook of my elbow to try and block out the scent. I hurried out of the room as fast as my legs could carry me, my heart pounding.

Once I escaped to an area where it felt a safe distance away, I gasped for a big breath of fresh, clean air. My body was intuitively trained to know what to do. I quickly found a nearby teacher to let her know what had happened. I'm sure she had already witnessed the commotion. It felt like minutes had gone by, but I'm sure it was only seconds.

As my nostrils grew hot, a tingling sensation engulfed me in a dizzying fog. I wondered if I was having an allergic reaction, all while keeping a close watch on myself as the teacher retrieved my bag of medications from my cubby.

I could feel each cell in my body pulsing rhythmically. Little did I understand my body was in the throes of a fight-or-flight response. I could practically hear the drumming of my pulse in my ears—*thump thump*—and the room seemed eerily quiet. Meanwhile, there was an intensity inside me that only I knew was being orchestrated. It's the same sensation I still experience when I catch a whiff of peanuts.

Trying to describe the sensation, it's as if a tiny bumble bee flew up my nostrils and started buzzing around. Within seconds, it triggers a tickling behind my eyes, zipping in circles before plunging down my throat and shooting to the tips of my toes. The concentrated energy leaves a trail of tiny electric currents, scorching everything in its wake. To this day, this is how I recognize the beginnings of an allergic reaction. It's not something I was ever explicitly taught; it's an innate awareness I've carried long before I even learned to read.

This particular "I SMELL PEANUT BUTTER" experience

left me with lip tingling and mild hives along the outer edges of my mouth. I was given a large swig of medicinal pink liquid, Children's Liquid Benadryl, leaving an unpleasant metallic bubblegum taste in my mouth.

A few years after this, I began to connect the dots about my allergy, piecing together that no one else in my circle of friends or family needed to check food labels for peanuts or peanut ingredients unless I was around. They turned to my family for answers, asking questions about my allergies instead of learning how to manage allergies themselves.

On top of that, I noticed their attitudes about eating were far different from my own heightened awareness. For me, there has never been any whimsy or freedom to eating, and certainly no food has gotten past me unstudied. In my 30s, I still approach every meal with caution—studying labels, scanning for hidden warnings, and smelling anything suspicious. It's a quiet ritual of survival, not trust.

Once the reaction subsided and I felt the reassuring sense that I'd be okay, a new feeling settled in: bewilderment. *How had peanuts made their way into my daycare?* It was time to channel my inner detective. Inspired by *Harriet the Spy* and *Mary-Kate and Ashley's Mystery* series, my Pre-K brain buzzed with curiosity. I was determined to crack the case of how something so dangerous ended up in someone's lunchbox. And thankfully not *my* lunchbox.

The same teacher who gave me my dose of liquid Benadryl expressed genuine concern about the incident, reassuring me my worries were valid. I breathed a sigh of relief, knowing they understood the dangers of peanut butter. Yet, I remained on high alert for days and weeks at preschool; truthfully, I haven't let my guard down since.

Later that week, I proudly informed the kids sitting near me at the long, rectangular lunch table that peanut butter was terrible stuff—not something to mess around with. I felt like the resident expert on the subject since I seemed to be the only kid at my preschool who knew about it. I was still riding the high of pride from speaking up earlier in the week, thinking I was protecting everyone. Little did I know, peanut butter was probably one of their favorite snacks!

Due to my life-threatening food allergy, my family didn't keep many, if any, peanut products in our home. I was taught that I was "severely allergic" from a young age. So, I intentionally hadn't been exposed to peanuts for this reason.

This early lunchtime memory was the first time I felt an allergic reaction come on without my mom by my side. While an allergic reaction doesn't always escalate to anaphylaxis, treating and monitoring it as if it could be is essential. Like most things, food allergies are a spectrum. Each person with a food allergy falls at a different point on the reactivity spectrum, and symptoms can vary widely with each reaction. There's no consistent formula or predictable pattern to follow.

I learned about the food allergy reactivity spectrum through Dr. Ruchi Gupta, her book, *Food Without Fear*, is my top book recommendation for anyone wanting to learn about food allergies or seeking validation for their own experiences. Dr. Gupta explains how reaction responses can change over time, making relying solely on past experiences as a guide impossible. It's also impossible to determine exactly how much of an allergen was ingested.

What might begin with seemingly minor symptoms can quickly escalate—resulting in facial swelling, throat tightness, itching around the neck, gastrointestinal distress, and potentially progressing to full-blown anaphylaxis.

The 2019 World Allergy Organization (WAO) Committee—part of a global network aligned with the World Health Organization (WHO)—defined anaphylaxis as "a serious systemic hypersensitivity reaction that is usually rapid in onset and may cause death. Severe anaphylaxis is characterized by potentially life-threatening compromise in airway, breathing and/or circulation, and may occur without typical skin features or circulatory shock being present."

While standardized definitions are crucial for diagnosis and treatment guidelines worldwide, they don't always align with how allergic reactions present in real life, especially in cases where symptoms are less textbook. This can lead to under-recognition and delayed administration of epinephrine.

It's also worth noting that the United States' relationship with the WHO has become politically fraught in recent years. The US was one of the 55 founding nations of the WHO in 1948, yet President Trump announced in January 2025 that the US would withdraw from the organization, with the withdrawal taking effect on January 22, 2026. A similar withdrawal was announced by Trump in 2020 but was later reversed by the Biden administration in 2021.

Why does this matter? Because when countries disengage from international health organizations, it can disrupt collaborative progress on global standards—including those for allergy diagnosis, research funding, and emergency response protocols.

Anaphylaxis is an acute and immediate reaction that demands prompt treatment, regardless of whether "typical" symptoms are present. In fact, about 10 to 20% of people experiencing anaphylaxis have no visible skin symptoms, such as hives or rash—symptoms many people (and even some medical professionals) expect to see. This lack of visible signs can contribute to delayed recognition and treatment. I've personally experienced this. In a recent anaphylactic episode, I didn't have the symptoms I had come to associate with the onset of a reaction—no hives on my face, no lip swelling. Instead, I was suddenly overwhelmed by a sense of doom and throat swelling. I knew the signs could vary, so I administered the epinephrine.

Dr. Farah Khan, a board-certified allergist with a social media presence, has previously shared helpful examples to illustrate how anaphylaxis can manifest across multiple systems of the body. Before seeing her content, I'd never seen anaphylaxis spelled out to this extent, and I found it personally so helpful for me to understand when to epi:

- Hives + vomiting = skin + gastrointestinal
- Lip swelling + coughing = skin + respiratory
- Itchy eyes + abdominal cramping = eyes + gastrointestinal
- Low blood pressure (dizziness) + hives = cardiovascular + skin
- Impending sense of doom + flushing = nervous system + skin

Since anaphylaxis occurs on a range, knowing when to use epinephrine isn't straightforward. Timing can feel tricky—using epinephrine too early, before symptoms clearly appear, might not address the peak of the reaction. However, delay can be dangerous. Allergy action plans made with a board-certified allergist can help guide decisions by emphasizing the importance of treating symptoms as they arise.

It's similar to when I first learned the science behind why baked goods can cause a delayed allergic response due to how the food protein breaks down more slowly when baked. For example, baked egg in something like a cupcake might cause a reaction a few hours later, whereas the same allergen could cause symptoms within a minute if it isn't baked.

One important takeaway I have for anyone who is dealing with a new diagnosis or newly learned topics, is to repeat your understanding back to your doctors, so they can confirm or clarify what you said before you leave the office. Your doctors should be approachable and willing to do this, as well as provide evidence-based answers you can revisit later to learn more. Asking my doctors about co-factors that can influence allergic reactions has helped me gain insight into how my body responds and why some of my reactions may look different at times. It's valuable to understand what co-factors can affect a reaction, such as hormones, alcohol, stress, illness, exercise, medications like NSAIDs, how a food is prepared, or how much allergen is present, especially at different stages of life from childhood through adulthood.

A common phrase is "Epi first, Epi fast," when there are clear signs of anaphylaxis. Even if there aren't multiple body systems engaged, if any one sign is rapidly progressing, it's suggested to use epinephrine than to not. No one feels eager to use epinephrine. Even the newer nasal formulations like Neffy come with hesitation—whether due to physical discomfort, anxiety, or financial concerns—but recognizing and responding to symptoms promptly can be the difference between life and death.

I can recall countless childhood memories tied to my peanut allergy, even ones that didn't involve an allergic reaction. For example, when everyone gathered for snack time, I'd be called over to sit beside the teacher. At first, I didn't mind—it felt like one-on-one attention. Can you tell I was an only child for 9 years? It made me feel special, as if I had my own little VIP seat.

Because of this part of my personality, it took a while for me to realize that the personal treatment was tied to my condition. Around first grade, age 6, a slow, self-conscious awareness started creeping in. I can't pinpoint the exact moment, but I began to resent the attention over time. I no longer wanted to sit apart or be singled out; I just wanted to blend in like everyone else in my friend group. This desire to fit in and to ignore my food allergy as much as possible lingered well into my teenage years and even early adulthood.

Over the years, my allergy has left me feeling isolated for various reasons. This still occasionally poses a challenge, though less so than when I was younger. It's a vulnerability I sometimes feel ashamed of—a part of me wishing I could blend in, not constantly needing to ask for accommodations or spend so much energy on what others consider simple tasks, like eating, drinking, or just being in communal spaces.

When people say, "I'm sorry," about my allergy, I usually respond with, "No, it's okay!" It's just one small part of who I am—like anyone living with a disability or chronic condition. The real frustration isn't from my allergy itself; it's the societal norms and lack of policies that create unnecessary barriers.

I also really appreciate the growing practice of using person-first language. For example, saying "a person with a disability" or "a person with a food allergy" instead of "disabled person" or "food-allergic person" emphasizes the humanness of anyone living with a condition. Not everyone prefers person-first language, but I see it as a thoughtful way to show respect and awareness. I'm still learning this myself, but I love the meaning behind it.

Navigating Childhood

I don't have any recollection of my earliest allergic reactions, so for the details of my first two, I've had to rely on family members to fill in the gaps. I know one happened at a small daycare where they were keeping me away from peanuts, but another child eating PB crackers nearby somehow contaminated me, and I broke out in a rash. The other occurred when I was two years old and my dad took me to Golden Gate Park, which was a regular part of my playtime routine growing up in San Francisco.

For those who don't know the context, food allergies were on the rise in the 1990s. Hence, the medical protocol was to avoid introducing peanuts, a common allergen, until children were older than 2. I was born with eczema on my hands, something my pediatrician identified as a potential indicator of food allergies in newborns. Because of this, my parents were told to be especially cautious with allergenic foods. But that day at the park, my dad gave me a cookie not realizing it contained peanut butter.

Afterward, my mom recalled noticing I was "acting funny,"

not quite myself, which prompted her to ask my dad what had happened. At first, she suspected I might have been stung by a bee. After asking a few questions, she inquired if I had eaten anything, and that's when my dad remembered the cookie that likely had peanut butter in it. From that point on, my parents were advised by my pediatrician to practice strict avoidance of my allergen—a precaution that, even as I write this, remains the primary treatment for those diagnosed with a food allergy today.

I didn't have another reaction to peanuts until I was on an airplane, of all places, flying from San Francisco to Louisville when I was 3 years old. I don't remember this vividly, but my mom has told me the story so many times it feels like I do. I begged her to let me smell one of the peanuts they handed everyone in those noisy, crinkly bags. She said I was so persistent that she hesitantly gave in, especially after I convinced her it didn't smell poisonous to me like it usually did. After that, I begged to taste it, and she apprehensively let me take the tiniest bite. She described it to me as a literal crumb, "just a lick of the corner." Immediately my mom could sense something was wrong, and it was obvious that I was still allergic.

Panic and regret set in as she swiftly grabbed for the Children's Liquid Benadryl. She always kept it handy and had me gulp it down in a rapid *glug glug glug*. Frantically, she waved down the flight attendants and asked for ice. Thankfully, I was okay, but that moment solidified for her that my peanut allergy likely wasn't going away. Though she regretted letting me have that tiny lick, as we all know, hindsight is 20/20—especially in the early '90s. Liquid Benadryl became a constant companion, sloshing around in my backpack throughout elementary school alongside my injectable epinephrine Jr.—the only treatment for life-threatening anaphylaxis.

At that time, I had a cousin who had recently outgrown their peanut allergy, which became a frequent topic in our extended family. They all assumed I would eventually follow suit. I was constantly asked, "Zoë, have you outgrown your peanut allergy yet?" And when I answered no, the response was always something like a confident, "Ah, well, you will." Sometimes, even, "Well, you will—have a peanut now to build up your immunity," which I definitely wouldn't do, and my parents were not on board with it either. Everyone outside of my immediate family seemed convinced of this outcome. Still, deep down, I had a gut feeling that my allergy wouldn't fade like my cousin's. Even at a young age, I sensed its potency.

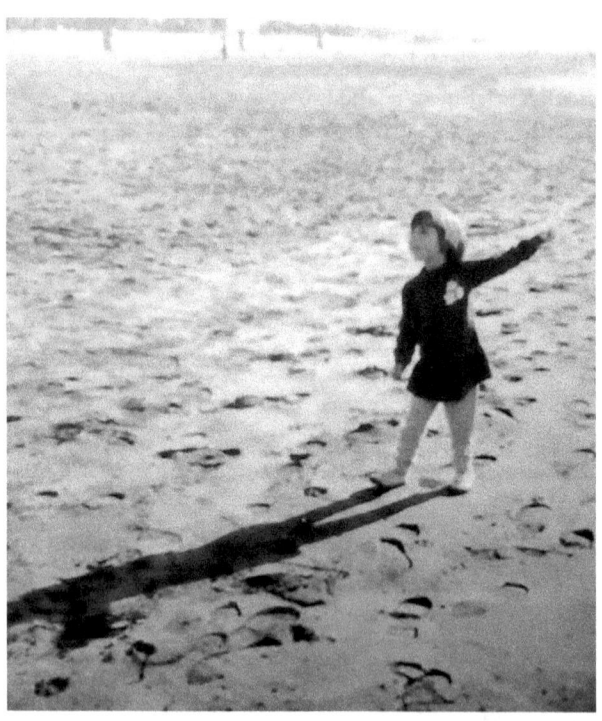

My parents never assumed I'd grow out of it, either. As I grew older and grasped the potential consequences of a reaction—namely, death—and could articulate my fears clearly, it hurt deeply that some of my family members didn't take my allergy seriously. I felt invalidated, which only added to my sense of shame about being different.

One family member repeatedly tried to give me peanuts, acting as if I chose to continue to have my allergy because I wouldn't eat small amounts. I was constantly looking over my shoulder, concerned that they might hide peanuts in my food when my parents or grandma, who took my allergy seriously, weren't looking. It wasn't out of malice, but I knew the potential consequences were poisonous, even at my young age. The seriousness of the situation created pressure to grow up faster and forced me to navigate complex fears and anxieties. I constantly monitored my environment in case someone slipped something into my food and learned that I couldn't trust all the adults around me.

Another early food allergy memory of mine takes me back to when I was about 8 years old, standing in our kitchen pantry at home as my mom sternly talked to my dad. Her voice echoed off the walls and down the hallway as she explained that he couldn't keep peanut butter in the house after he attempted to make a PB&J sandwich. Hearing the words "peanut butter" instantly captured my full attention and heightened my anxiety. It was as if an antenna had popped up from my mind, immediately alerting me.

Later that evening, I crept into the pantry, the soft creak of the door amplifying the quiet tension of the moment. My eyes roamed over the shelves, scanning, searching, and lingering on jars and boxes until they landed on it. There it was. A jar perched high on the top shelf, just out of reach, its label partially obscured by the shadows. I stood frozen, staring at it, my thoughts a tangle of unease. Part of me wanted to throw it away to erase the worry it brought but instead I gently closed the pantry door and walked back to my room with a heavy knot of uncertainty twisting in my chest. I wasn't sure what to feel—fear, sadness, or something else entirely—and that confusion settled over me like a shadow.

My mom had always warned me how dangerous peanuts were for my health, so I didn't understand why my dad didn't seem to take the same care. He wanted to have peanuts in our home even though he knew they could hurt me. My mind buzzed with questions about food allergies long before Google was around. I wondered, *Could peanuts hurt my dad?* and *Why would anyone want to eat something that might hurt others?*

I thought back to how I sensed my mom's anger and worry in her raised voice, crossed arms, and furrowed brow. In contrast, my dad looked bewildered, his hands in the air, clearly not getting it. He walked away, indifferent to the tension, his footsteps a rhythmic stomping. If my memory serves me right, this was one of many times she threw his peanut butter away, only for him to retrieve it from the trash later or buy a new jar to replace it.

My main takeaway from these interactions of witnessing the tossing and repurchasing of peanut butter was the unsettling realization that I couldn't fully trust my dad when it came to my allergy. I never understood what was so special about peanut butter that it needed to be in our home. This feeling mirrored countless moments when I felt less important than an optional food item. Being relegated to a position of lesser value due to my food allergy stirred up a whirlwind of emotions, including shame, which left me feeling vulnerable. I internalized this, often feeling misunderstood, heightening my need to constantly ensure my own safety without relying on others.

My advice for raising children with food allergies is for parents to be mindful of their words and actions, as they can have a profound emotional impact, as I experienced firsthand. My relationship with my father was good at times but also tumultuous throughout my upbringing, and in hindsight, small moments like these undoubtedly contributed. As a child, I didn't have the words to explain how his actions made me feel, or how much I longed for him to see that my daily needs mattered—that I mattered more than food. At the time, I assumed he just wasn't empathetic, but now I understand that he is; I simply didn't have the words to express myself back then. Those feelings stayed buried inside me for decades, only coming to the surface when I began unpacking them in therapy as an adult.

My dad has a food allergy of his own, a likely non–IgE-mediated reaction to cantaloupe, which he has managed on his own without formal testing. This means the reaction doesn't involve his immune system in the typical allergic way, but it does cause gastrointestinal issues. His reactions differ from my peanut allergy, which is IgE-mediated, because my reactions involve my immune system and multiple organ systems, posing immediate life-threatening risks. Understanding this context of IgE and non–IgE helps me grasp why he and others in my life sometimes seemed to think I was overreacting in managing my allergy. It simply wasn't within their range of experience, so their understanding was limited, at least until they saw the reality for themselves.

Now, as an adult, I can empathize with my dad's perspective to an extent. I'm not excusing his lack of awareness because his attitude was deeply impactful. However, wearing my empathetic hat, I recognize that I was his first child, and navigating a life-threatening food allergy was uncharted territory for him. We didn't have access to knowledgeable allergists or the vast number of resources on the internet as we do now. The recent experience with my cousin outgrowing their peanut allergy also likely influenced his actions.

Funnily enough, my childhood best friend also had a peanut allergy. Proving how different reactivity can be, her main symptom from peanut ingestion was hyperactivity, which was similar to my cousin's response before he outgrew his. It's a stark reminder that food allergies and reactions defy generalization—each person's experience is their unique food allergy reactivity fingerprint, in a sense.

Over time, I've learned to accept that I don't need everyone to validate my food allergy experience, and that realization has been incredibly freeing. As I grew up, my support system expanded beyond just my family—my friends also became an important source of support. I'm fortunate to now have an even more extensive network that includes online friends around the globe, colleagues, family, a trusted allergist, friends, and my husband, who is always prepared to monitor my symptoms and administer my epinephrine on me if needed. And now, my dad and I have repaired our relationship—he is considerate, trusts my words, and takes my allergy seriously.

At the end of the day, what matters most is my own self-compassion and validation of my allergy experience. For those managing food allergies, or caring for someone who is, I believe in empowering the allergic person to advocate for themselves. As much as I appreciate having friends and family who are willing to administer my epinephrine and watch for my symptoms, I also need to know how to handle it on my own. I recently experienced anaphylaxis while traveling alone, hours away from home. Being able to clearly communicate with strangers around me and confidently use my epinephrine was life-saving, and everything worked out.

Clear communication is key to ensuring food allergy safety. And while having allies to advocate alongside you is invaluable, not everyone will be open to learning or willing to accommodate. I've stopped wasting energy trying to convince people to care—because honestly, having food allergies is an incredible radar for figuring out who deserves a spot in your inner circle. The way someone responds says everything about whether they're someone I want to keep close.

As uncomfortable as it can be to learn to advocate for yourself, it's essential. No one can read your mind to know what you're allergic to, whether it's IgE or non-IgE-mediated, what to do in the event of a reaction, if you have epinephrine on you, or how your symptoms may present. Some allergic reactions are triggered not only by ingestion but also by exercise after eating certain foods—known as exercise-induced food allergies—which can cause symptoms similar to other allergic reactions. This is where the invisible nature of food allergies becomes especially important—it takes clear communication to express your needs and accommodation preferences.

Today, cross-contact remains the primary cause of my allergic reactions, made worse by the inadequate food label transparency in the United States. *Sniff, sniff* was the soundtrack of my childhood, and in many ways, it still is. I've always relied on my nose to help detect whether peanuts are present in an environment or hidden in a product. My early years were a blend of ordinary childhood joys tempered by an ever-present intensity of caution. Surprisingly, my mom insists it wasn't as stressful as one might imagine. And from my memory, I agree with her; I don't recall feeling particularly stressed about it as a child. It was simply the reality and hand I was dealt, and we managed it together.

My peanut allergy has undeniably shaped my life from an early age and had a big impact on my parents' experience as first-time parents, figuring out how to manage food allergies before smartphones existed and before most people even had dial-up internet. My family and I became experts at navigating a world full of hidden dangers—meticulously reading labels, asking questions, staying vigilant about our surroundings, and always having emergency medication on hand.

Over time, I've learned that food allergies aren't just triggered by ingestion. Research by the NIH and the Allergy & Asthma Network shows that food proteins can become airborne during cooking processes, like steaming and boiling. I've personally experienced reactions from saliva becoming airborne when someone spoke to me after recently consuming peanut butter. It may seem obvious, but dust or residue from allergens on shared surfaces can also trigger allergic reactions. Just like pollen in the air can make us sneeze or cause other symptoms, airborne food proteins can affect those of us with food allergies in similar ways.

Imagine someone shaking a bag of roasted peanuts into their hand. The dust can spread beyond their skin, landing on their clothing or surrounding areas and on anything they touch next before washing their hands—a door, steering wheel, their phone, their keys. These examples highlight that exposure risks go far beyond direct ingestion and reinforce the importance of awareness in environments where allergens may be present in less obvious ways. Someone might put their phone away or drive someplace and then wash their hands, but those surfaces can continue to re-contaminate until they're properly cleaned.

My journey is a testament to perseverance, adapting and evolving to unpredictability, and not living in fear. It's about living a rich, fulfilling life despite the constraints imposed by food allergies. This narrative isn't solely mine. There are countless individuals and families who have transformed their food allergy experiences into sources of inspiration and opportunities for change.

The family behind Elijah's Law and the Elijah-Alavi Foundation (EAF) have become a powerful voice for food allergy awareness, advocating for safer school and child care environments after the tragic loss of their 3-year-old son, Elijah, to a fatal anaphylactic reaction after being given his allergen at daycare. In his memory, Elijah's Law requires all child care facilities to follow specific guidelines to prevent, recognize, and respond to life-threatening allergic reactions.

Recently, the family behind the SB 68 ADDE Act has been working to mandate allergen labeling on restaurant menus in California. I'm thrilled to announce, it passed and was signed into law, and is the first bill of its kind in the US requiring large restaurant chains (20+ locations nationwide) to clearly disclose the top 9 allergens on their menus in the state of California. By contrast, all restaurants in the EU—big and small—have been required to provide this information since 2014, with no size-based exceptions.

Similarly, Lianne Mandelbaum, founder of the non-profit, The No Nut Traveler, tirelessly campaigns for safer air travel for those with food allergies, addressing ongoing airline issues that continue to significantly impact the food allergy community. Lastly, I'd be remiss if I didn't recognize Amanda Orlando, who continues to pave the way through honest and authentic conversations in the food allergy space. In the May 2025 issue of *Allergic Living* magazine, Amanda published a powerful article titled "Women with Food Allergies: Why Many Are Afraid to Get Pregnant." In it, she writes:

> *Patient advocacy for parents of kids with food allergies focuses helpfully on information so that parents can make educated decisions. However, what about the large cohort of millennials who have food allergies themselves and are of parenting age? Yes, those of us who were part of the first big wave of allergic kids are now having children. Yet for this journey, there are little to no resources to guide us.*

This resonated deeply with me as I've carried that exact fear. It likely influenced my thinking when I was younger and may have played a part in my decision of not wanting kids early on. I now wonder if I unconsciously ruled out parenthood because of my allergy—fearing how I'd navigate cross-contact with a child eating allergens, or how I could safely be present at school events and birthday parties.

We're now openly approaching questions like: How would I introduce food allergens in a way that's safe for kids and for me? What do I do when my child inevitably comes home from daycare or a friend's house carrying traces of my allergen on their skin or clothes? These are complex, emotional questions without easy answers. These conversations are happening more often now, thanks to leaders like Amanda who are naming the realities many of us quietly carry. As we continue to raise our voices and ask hard questions, we're also helping to build a more inclusive, supportive future for people with food allergies.

Their stories, like mine, echo the power of resilience and the transformation of adversity into advocacy. They remind me that while food allergies present unique challenges, they also foster communities that are supportive, compassionate, and open-minded. Personally, I've found that advocacy has been deeply healing for my mental health—creating a sense of collective connection and reminding me that I'm not alone. It's empowering to know that by sharing my experiences, I'm not only helping myself but also making a difference in others' lives. I aspire to illuminate the incredible work being done in this space, creating a vibrant tapestry of awareness that encourages people to live fully and fearlessly.

Advocacy can look different for everyone. For some, it's public speaking, policy change, or organizing events. For others, it's storytelling, art, or simply navigating daily life with integrity and intention. When I first met my partner, he told me, "You vote with your dollars." I had never heard that phrase before, and it honestly changed the way I thought about everyday choices.

At the time, I was shopping at places that didn't align with my values, and he gently pointed that out. It was a small moment that opened me up to advocacy in a whole new way. Now I see that where we choose—or choose not—to spend our money is its own powerful form of activism. As a food allergy community, we have the ability to support brands that care about safety and inclusion, and to withhold support from those that don't. Every decision we make, no matter how quiet or personal, has the potential to ripple outward and help build a more thoughtful world.

Closing Thoughts & Additional Context

- Prevalence of Food Allergies: According to FARE (Food Allergy Research & Education), as of 2024, 33 million Americans, including 1 in 10 adults and 1 in 13 children (roughly two children per classroom), have at least one food allergy. Alarmingly, more than 40% of children with food allergies and over 51% of adults have experienced severe reactions. Nearly 11% of adults aged 18 or older have at least one food allergy, underscoring the magnitude of this issue. These figures likely underrepresent the true prevalence due to unreported cases stemming from limited healthcare access and inadequate food allergy education.

- Eczema and the "Atopic March": Eczema, asthma, and food allergies are three related inflammatory conditions known as the *atopic march*. Only in adulthood did I learn about the connection between eczema and food allergies—when eczema flares, the skin barrier becomes compromised, which may allow allergens from the environment or food to penetrate the skin, interacting with immune cells, and mistakenly viewed as immune threats. This is why treating eczema and keeping the skin healthy, especially in babies, is so important. While the exact cause of food allergies remains unknown, protecting and healing the skin barrier is believed to play a crucial role in prevention.

- Overlooked Needs: As we continue to explore the many stages of life where food allergies are often misunderstood or under-supported, it's also vital to consider the intersection of food allergies with other disabilities—both visible and invisible. For individuals who are neurodivergent, including those with autism or intellectual disabilities, or those living with physical or cognitive impairments, the need for advocacy can be even greater. Communicating about allergies, understanding complex ingredient labels, or asserting boundaries in shared environments may not always be possible without support. And yet, these individuals face the same risks and deserve the same protections. In these cases, a caregiver, family member, or trained advocate plays a critical role—not just in safety, but in dignity and autonomy. It raises the question: how are we ensuring that these voices are being heard and these needs respected? In a society where access and inclusion are still catching up, people who require assistance with daily living also need assistance navigating the complexities of food allergy management. We can't assume self-advocacy is always an option—and we must do better to create systems that account for that.

- Modes of Exposure: Food allergies can be triggered not only through ingestion but also through exposure to allergens on contaminated surfaces or in airborne particles. Cross-contact with allergenic dust and proteins, whether on surfaces or in the air, is common and difficult to track due to its microscopic nature.

- A Shift in Allergy Prevention Strategies: In the 1990s, the medical field advised parents to avoid introducing top food allergens to children at risk of allergies. However, it became evident that this approach inadvertently contributed to the rise in food allergy cases. Current research now promotes the early introduction of allergens as a preventive measure, encouraging resilience against allergies from infancy. This shift in strategy highlights our evolving understanding that early exposure can help lower the risk of developing food allergies. In 2015 the LEAP study (Learning Early About Peanut Allergy), published in the *New England Journal of Medicine*, demonstrated that introducing peanut products to high-risk infants could significantly reduce the likelihood of developing peanut allergy. Now nearly a decade later new real-world population data confirms what the study predicted: feeding babies peanut early and consistently has helped thousands of children avoid peanut allergy in the first place.

- Limitations and Realities: Of course this does not apply to every allergy. Alpha-gal syndrome, for example, develops later in life after a tick bite, and adult-onset food allergies in general are rising. There are also families who were following medical guidance in the 1990s and 2000s to avoid allergenic foods during infancy and later developed allergies, which carries its own heartbreak. And even when families do everything "right" and follow early-introduction guidelines, some children still develop food allergies anyway. But it is encouraging to know that current guidance is backed by research and offers one evidence-based route that may reduce risk for many.

- IgE vs. Non–IgE Allergies: Food allergies are categorized into IgE-mediated and non–IgE-mediated types. IgE allergies trigger a rapid immune response to specific food allergens, leading to immediate and potentially life-threatening reactions like anaphylaxis. Common symptoms include hives, swelling, difficulty breathing, and anaphylaxis. On the other hand, non–IgE allergies involve delayed immune responses, often occurring hours or days later, and can lead to disruptions in daily life without invoking the immune system's immediate response. These reactions commonly manifest as gastrointestinal issues and inflammation. Cow's milk and gluten are among the most common non–IgE allergens. Diagnosis typically involves a strict 4-6 week elimination diet to test for sensitivities, and are often linked to conditions like eosinophilic esophagitis (EoE) and food protein-induced enterocolitis syndrome (FPIES). I recommend the CURED Foundation as a resource for EoE, and for FPIES, The FPIES Foundation—great places to learn more if you want additional information.

- MCAS and the Evolving Allergy Landscape: I'd be remiss

not to mention MCAS, or mast cell activation syndrome, a condition that's becoming more widely recognized in the allergy community. Mast cells are part of the immune system, and in MCAS they can release chemicals inappropriately or too easily, causing a wide range of symptoms: hives, flushing, gastrointestinal distress, low blood pressure, a rapid heartbeat, or even anaphylaxis. Diagnosis can be complicated, often taking several years and multiple specialists, because the symptom picture overlaps with so many other conditions. It's also important to note that not every condition that gets grouped in with "food allergy" is actually an IgE-mediated allergy. For example, celiac disease is an autoimmune disease that is primarily IgA-mediated. Gluten triggers an immune attack on the body's own small intestine. It is not a food allergy, even though it requires meticulous avoidance—but the consequences, the language, and the daily precautions often sit in the same universe. Just as food allergies have become more widely understood over the past decade, MCAS is just beginning to enter mainstream awareness, and I imagine it will continue to be talked about much more in the coming years. I'm looking into this myself as a possible diagnosis right now, because I'm experiencing an overlap of symptoms that makes MCAS a realistic possibility. For reliable, in-depth information and education on MCAS, The Mast Cell Disease Society (TMS) offers a trusted starting point.

- Resources for Further Information: Diagnosing a food allergy is a complex process. Over 100 million Americans have allergic conditions, and more than 33 million of those have food allergies. To stay informed about the latest recommendations regarding food allergy prevention and research for treatments and a cure, resources such as the Food Allergy & Anaphylaxis Connection Team (FAACT), the Center for Food Allergy & Asthma Research (CFAAR), the Asthma and Allergy

Foundation of America (AAFA), and the Food Allergy Science Initiative (FASI) continue to offer valuable, reliable, and current insight. And of course, seeing a board-certified allergist is key—they can provide personalized guidance, confirm diagnoses, and help you develop a management plan.

2

MIDDLE & HIGH SCHOOL YEARS

High School

It was a gray, dreary day. The school hallways were so dimly lit they looked foggy, a grayscale dance of varying lights and shadows as I walked to my first-period class. The weather matched my sleepy mood as I approached the English 101 door, so much so that I began to appreciate the relief of the monochromatic hallways compared to the artificial sunbeam pouring out from the bright room I was advancing on.

Squinting hard as I entered, I stepped over the threshold into the harsh, intrusive glare of fluorescent lights. My ears flinched at the sudden startle from a bunch of competing, unruly voices, the chorus of a nearly full classroom. Two words: sensory overload. It was barely 9 a.m.

Having just turned 15, it was the middle of my freshman year. For my recent birthday, my friends surprised me by filling my locker with tons of small balloons, a gesture I absolutely loved. My school was small, encompassing grades K–12, with fewer than 500 students. It was public, but you had to apply to attend, and they accepted based on the fulfilling diversity of zip codes.

The whole school felt like a close-knit community. I was fortunate to get in during 7th grade, but adjusting was challenging as the only new student that year. I felt like an outsider among students who had grown up together from kindergarten, especially when some of the girls who I'd hoped to befriend expressed disappointment that I wasn't a "cute boy" on my first day.

By my freshman year, I had settled in after two years at the school. I was no longer the new kid, and the new students brought fresh dynamics and excitement to the existing class. On the first day of school, I met Teah in math class and gave her a fair warning: I was terrible at math, so if she wanted to sit with others at a different table, I completely understood. To my surprise, she admitted she wasn't great at math either and eagerly chose to sit beside me instead. She remains one of my closest friends to this day.

While I had friends from earlier grades, I was open to forming new connections. Throughout my school years, I never quite fit into a single group; instead, I always connected with different circles and tended to act as a social bridge between cliques.

Alana was one of my closest school friends from 7th and 8th grade. I frequently stayed overnight at her house, bonding with her parents and two younger brothers. They treated me as an honorary fourth sibling, and I joined them for many family events. However, as freshman year began, we organically started to drift apart. Our once-frequent talks and hangouts gradually happened less often.

Despite this, we remained on good terms. Alana knew everything about me, from my family dynamics at home to my peanut allergy. I trusted her completely, thinking I could rely on her for anything, just as she could me, so what happened next shattered our bond and deeply betrayed me in this formative period.

That same murky winter day during freshman year, when I walked into the overly bright English 101 class, I was utterly blindsided, in a different way, by what transpired. Alana and a few of her friends were standing in a circle on the room's right-hand side. Usually, I would head left to join Teah, Lux, and Brian at our usual table. But that day, on a whim, I decided to turn right and join Alana's group until class started. She had an unusual, mischievous grin while casually snacking from a small plastic bag, chewing slowly. Her eyes fixed on me as I approached.

"Hey Alana, what's up?" I smiled and waved. Instead of replying, she extended a friendly invitation to try some of her snacks. Wrongly assuming they were safe, I said, "Thanks, what is it?" and reached into the bag curiously. Her grin widened, reassuring me that it couldn't possibly contain peanuts—after all, she knew about my allergy. She was acting a bit strange, but I brushed it off, thinking she wouldn't risk giving me something unsafe regardless.

"Wait, but what is it?" I asked again, chuckling and pondering what it could be. Then, more directly, I asked, "Does it have peanuts?" Alana just replied in a cryptic voice, "Try it and see."

In hindsight, that should've tipped me off! But I honestly didn't think a close friend would ever put my life at risk. Especially after no major falling-out happened between us. Alana had a very different sense of humor than I did, so I assumed she was joking and cautiously sniffed the small round puff. It smelled odd but not exactly like peanuts to me. Based on the smell, I wondered if it was something with sesame. This incident stands as the only time my peanut-sensitive nose led me astray.

I placed a single round puff on my tongue and instantly recognized the presence of peanuts. My face went slack, eyes wide. I spat it out onto the floor, scratching at my tongue to try and remove any residue. Panic set in; my heavy backpack suddenly felt like a huge burden. Flinging it across the floor, I sprinted into the hallway, racing for the nearby bathroom sink. I frantically scooped water from the sink into my mouth and repeatedly spit it out.

As I mentally mapped out my location in the U-shaped building, I realized I was the farthest point from the school office, where my life-saving medication was required by school policy to be kept locked away. I quickly grasped the extreme inconvenience—and the potential danger—of being so distant. *Could I even reach it in time?* I wondered, but I knew I had to try.

Growing up asthmatic hadn't conditioned my body for this. I'd never run a mile without getting a side cramp, let alone without giving up halfway. In gym class, I'd been known to dramatically hop on a track runner's back to finish the last half mile or just downright refuse to run. My face turns beet red at the first signs of any physical activity; it's how I've always been. Despite this, I bolted as fast as I could down three flights of stairs, through the hallways, and catapulted myself into the school office, clutching my throat. Pointing inside my mouth, I screamed, "I ate a peanut! I need my medicine!"

Everyone at the school knew me as "the one with the peanut allergy," so there was no mistaking the urgency. They quickly gave me my liquid Benadryl and put my epinephrine pens beside me. I chugged the liquid medicine, too afraid to use my epinephrine injector right away. I opted to monitor my symptoms first since I hadn't ingested the cereal puff but only touched my tongue to it.

When they called my mom, I quickly explained what had happened. She arrived in a flurry, undoubtedly alarmed and perplexed by the situation. My mom understood my vigilance around my allergy; she knew I took it more seriously than anyone, so this whole situation seemed suspicious to her.

I was too embarrassed to return to my classroom to retrieve my backpack, not wanting to face Alana, so I asked the office aide to grab it. Thankfully, I was fine, and my symptoms didn't last beyond the day. I lived to tell the tale this time but still was in disbelief that I almost ate a piece of Reese's Puffs cereal. Why Alana cattily gave it to me, knowing it was Reese's Puffs, I don't know. She never apologized or mentioned it, so I never mentioned it to her, either. I was waiting for her to apologize, and the absence of acknowledgment from her spoke volumes to the point where I no longer considered her my friend.

Meanwhile, the table I usually sat with in class witnessed the exchange go down from afar. They were blowing up my phone to try to find out if I was okay and the details of what happened. After I told them, none of us could wrap our minds around the headspace Alana was in to give me something deadly. It made me feel better that they were equally as slighted and confused. My mind flooded with recent memories of Alana's family's church camp being kept peanut-free on the days I attended, and how her parents went out of their way to make me safe meals and snacks during slumber parties just a year before this incident.

Adding a bitter twist to the anguish, Alana was one of the few with an intimate understanding of my allergy. She understood my challenges around speaking up for myself and how I felt socially isolated due to it—at least, I'd thought she did. *Did I, perhaps, misinterpret our friendship? Did I do something to her that made her want to... end me?* The unspoken question is still there nearly two decades later.

The haunting memory of her deceptive smile still lingers in my mind, woven with the image of her allowing me to reach into the bag without stopping me. After that incident, my mom made me keep my medications in my backpack, going against the school policy. To do so, my family spent additional money out of pocket to get more epinephrine so that I'd have enough for a 2-pack in the school office, satisfying their need to have it locked away, and an additional 2-pack in my backpack. I confided in my mom about how sad and frustrated I was with Alana for putting me in that situation and how I didn't know what to do. The weight of it left me raw and shaky, like I had nowhere else to put the hurt. My mom reassured me and validated my experience, giving me a long hug and reminding me how glad she was that I was safe.

Over the years, I've experienced the joy of making it through a day without a reaction. It may sound amusing to celebrate a lack of reaction, but it comes from the highly contrasting memories of sheer terror when I've been faced with an unexpected one.

Each event or gathering I've attended as far back as I can remember has required me to mention my allergy and maintain a level of attentiveness. An uncommunicated change or something unexpected can instantly turn a simple moment into a potentially stressful environment. Thankfully, even past romantic partners who may have acted "too cool" or fallen short in other ways always took my peanut allergy seriously.

I've been fortunate in this aspect, knowing that those who truly grasp the severity of my condition have been my anchors. Their empathy and efforts to help create safe spaces for me have enabled me to engage more fully in life despite the very real, constant risk of anaphylaxis. I didn't have the same robust and supportive social network in middle and high school as I do now. Unfortunately, the experience of having my allergen given to me on purpose by Alana wasn't the only uncomfortable moment I faced at school. Still, it remains the most traumatic and malicious one.

A year or so later, my close friend Sally caught me off guard between classes one day when she asked if I ever worried about how easy it would be for someone to kill me. Her question stunned me, focusing on the word *kill* she used. She casually followed up with a matter-of-fact tone, "Well, someone could slip a peanut into your sandwich without you knowing, and it couldn't be traced back to them, you know?" as she handed me my packed lunchbox from the school fridge. It's been over 15 years, and I still dwell on that comment. I remember holding my sandwich, questioning whether she was trying to convey a hint.

"Should I not eat this?" I asked, and she assured me it was just a hypothetical, passing comment. I was left unable to shake the unease it left behind. Despite my anxiety, I ate the sandwich, and thankfully, everything was fine. Yet, from that moment on, a seed of doubt took root within me, which had never existed in my relationship with her before.

Middle School

Regarding food allergy bullying, an earlier memory from the year I was in sixth grade comes to mind. It involves my orchestra teacher, a person I had previously found absolutely hilarious and admired. That was until he caught me off guard by unexpectedly targeting my peanut allergy.

In what should have been a nurturing classroom environment, my orchestra teacher unexpectedly bestowed upon me the unwelcome nickname "Goober," a slang word for peanut. Since he knew I had a peanut allergy, he explained the meaning to me as he called me that, and then repeated it frequently. It wasn't just a one-off comment; it felt like he was determined to work the word "Goober" into every conversation, saying it loudly and boisterously for everyone to hear. While some might have seen it as slightly endearing, it felt like a jab to me. This new label, which I'd never heard before he explained it, combined with all eyes on me in class, felt like a weight pulling me down.

After a few weeks of this, I knew I had to say something. I rehearsed what I planned to say repeatedly, preparing myself to confront him about the nickname in private after class. I found it particularly anxiety-inducing since I had already engaged in multiple discussions with him that year about how peanut-containing snacks were being eaten in the classroom. Given that context, his use of the nickname felt like a mocking acknowledgment of my allergy, belittling me.

After class let out one day, I summoned the courage to casually mention it to him in the hall when no other students were around. This was a feat in itself since he was popular, and students often stayed after to talk with him.

I calmly told him I knew it likely came from a kind place, but that I disliked the nickname "Goober," and I pointed out its meaning. Instead of reconsidering, he doubled down, encouraging others nearby in the hallway to call me it, even chanting it at me. At only 11 years old, I knew this was an inappropriate reaction from someone who was supposed to have my best interest in mind. My defenses went up, and for the rest of the year, I played my instrument quietly, shrinking into the background of the classroom, just hoping the teacher wouldn't call me it again.

Throughout elementary and middle school, even into early high school, if I felt a reaction starting or my stomach was acting up, I'd quietly excuse myself to the bathroom without saying a word to anyone. I didn't want anyone to follow me in or ask questions; I just wanted privacy and to avoid any extra attention. I didn't carry my medicine with me back then, and no one ever knew what I was dealing with or why I'd suddenly disappear.

Looking back, I realize how dangerous that was. I know it's common at that age to feel shy or hesitant to speak up about something so personal, but if you're managing a life-threatening allergy yourself or for your child or family member, this is exactly the kind of thing to talk about openly with people you trust. Even something as simple as practicing a short sentence—like "I'm not feeling well, can you come with me?"—can make it easier to speak up instead of silently slipping away.

Always keeping your medicine on you is crucial—even if it was or is against school policy! I say, break it. Your safety is more important than a rule made by someone who doesn't fully understand the risks. Even with your medicine on you, if something were to happen behind a closed bathroom door, no one would know to check. It's not worth risking your life over the fear of a little embarrassment—especially in a space everyone ends up in eventually! And that teacher making fun of me? It just goes to show that joking about allergic reactions or symptoms isn't funny, it's harmful. It teaches people to stay quiet when speaking up could save their lives.

Closing Thoughts & Additional Context

- The Importance of Support Systems: Strong support systems—like therapy, community groups, and friendships—are vital for handling the emotional ups and downs of food allergies. These networks provide practical help and understanding, creating a sense of safety in everyday life. Therapy can help you work through anxiety, while support groups allow you to share experiences with others who get it. Building relationships with people who respect your needs can truly transform your journey, giving you the confidence to face challenges with more resilience.

- Bullying: According to a survey by FARE (Food Allergy Research & Education), approximately one-third of kids, or 1 in 3 kids with food allergies, report being bullied due to their food allergy condition. This is particularly serious because if a bully exposes someone to their allergen, it can lead to life-threatening consequences. FARE, along with the Food Allergy & Anaphylaxis Connection Team (FAACT) and Kids with Food Allergies (KFA)—the food allergy division of the Asthma and Allergy Foundation of America (AAFA)—offer resources and education on food allergy bullying prevention through their websites to help raise awareness and promote safety.

- School Bullying Policies: School bullying policies vary, but their effectiveness often depends on a school's commitment to inclusivity and proactive engagement from administrators. Schools should implement policies emphasizing empathy, inclusivity, and respect for differences to reduce bullying. Engaging with students at risk of bullying is one way a school can be proactive. Asking open-ended questions to someone you suspect may be getting bullied can also help identify issues. Examples of these questions include: "Have you felt safe and comfortable at school recently?" "Is there anyone who has made you feel excluded?" "Do you feel that you are treated differently because of your health concerns?" and "Has anything at school made you feel threatened or left out?" These questions should be directed to students, but they can also be shared with teachers, counselors, or the school principal, since those adults are often responsible for identifying bullying and enforcing policies. And of course, these questions can apply to all children in settings beyond school as well.

- FAACT School Education Resources: FAACT offers a comprehensive range of free K-12 educational resources for teachers, parents, and schools to help students understand food allergies and anaphylaxis. Their Food Allergy Curricula Program for Schools provides age-appropriate lesson plans, interactive activities, and teacher-designed PowerPoint presentations for every grade level. Each includes certificates for students, perfect for Food Allergy Awareness Month in May and beyond. While aligning with CDC guidelines, the programs are flexible for classroom adaptation, continually updated, and easy to download from FAACT's website, allowing educators to share these invaluable resources widely.

- Medication Accessibility: Life-saving medications like epinephrine should be kept physically on or close to the allergic person, whether in a purse, bag, or pocket. Needle-injector epinephrine can degrade in high temperatures, so it's important to follow storage guidelines and use insulated carrying cases during warmer months to ensure the medication remains effective. While nasal spray versions like Neffy offer greater temperature tolerance, monitoring temperatures carefully, as detailed on the packaging, is still essential to maintain efficacy.

- Section 504 Plans: Section 504 Plans, now widely implemented in US K-12 schools, recognize food allergies as valid disabilities and provide essential support through emergency protocols and written documentation tailored to students with food allergies. This represents significant progress in food allergy awareness and management. When I was in school, such plans weren't available, but today, they've become a standardized tool for ensuring student safety, accommodation, and inclusion.

- Legal Challenges to Section 504: In September 2024, a coalition of 17 states filed a lawsuit—Texas v. Becerra—challenging the US Department of Health and Human Services' (HHS) updated regulations under Section 504 of the Rehabilitation Act. These updates were designed to strengthen protections for individuals with disabilities, including students with food allergies. The lawsuit not only seeks to roll back these new protections but also, in a more extreme move, questions the constitutionality of Section 504 itself. Even if your state is not directly involved, this case carries significant national implications and is worth watching closely.

- Rising Threats to Section 504 Protections: In early 2025, disability advocates raised serious concerns about efforts by the current US administration to weaken the enforcement of civil rights protections under 504. As discussed on a recent podcast episode of *Don't Feed the Fear* featuring attorney Laurel Francoeur, changes are happening through executive actions—cutting funding and capacity in key departments like the Department of Justice and the Office for Civil Rights. This is especially alarming because discrimination cases involving 504 violations are already being dismissed at the federal level, leaving students—whether they have food allergies, chronic illnesses, or are part of the trans community—vulnerable and unprotected. While some states have anti-discrimination laws, most only have enforcement mechanisms for IEPs, not 504 Plans. It's a troubling shift that signals a broader deprioritization of disability rights, racial equity, and gender inclusion in schools. As families, we can still contact our state's Attorney General to push back, and organizations like FAACT are continuing to share stories of how 504 protections have made a real difference. But the reality is: *the fight for disability rights is far from over—and it affects all of us.*

- Executive Actions and DEI Rollbacks: In addition to these legal challenges, 2025 saw executive actions that further weakened civil rights and DEI initiatives at the federal level. On January 21, Executive Order 14173 revoked affirmative action requirements for federal contractors and curtailed federal DEI programs, while key offices promoting equity and inclusion faced cuts or closure. Advocates warn these moves signal a broader deprioritization of protections for marginalized communities—including individuals with disabilities—making it even harder to ensure safe, inclusive environments.

- Check Out *ImmuniForce: The Anaphylaxis Strike*: A first-of-its-kind graphic novel recently released for the food allergy and asthma communities—and beyond. The story follows a team of superheroes dedicated to protecting people from food allergies and asthma-related emergencies. Co-founded by Thomas Silvera of the Elijah-Alavi Foundation, it was published in 2025 and is perfect for ages 6 to 15 and up. As an adult, I enjoyed it too. It's an engaging, action-packed story that teaches kids about safety, awareness, and the power of teamwork.

- Peanut Allergy Disability: In the US, the ADA (Americans with Disabilities Act) recognizes food allergies as a valid disability. This means that food allergies should be accepted as a disability, and that designation should not be questioned when someone identifies as having a food allergy disability and requires accommodations. While not everyone with a food allergy considers it a disability, some do, depending on where they fall on the reactivity spectrum. With the 2008 passing of the ADA Amendments Act (ADAAA), food allergies began to be recognized as applicable disabilities. The amendments broadened the definition of what constitutes a disability, specifically including conditions like food allergies, where the body's immune response to certain foods can substantially limit major life activities, such as eating or breathing. This clarification ensures that individuals with food allergies are entitled to reasonable accommodations in various settings, including schools and workplaces.

3

COLLEGE AND EARLY 20S

Airborne Allergic

Throughout my life, I've been able to sense peanut particles in the air. Despite multiple allergists insisting to me that being "airborne allergic" was impossible, I deduced they were wrong. My body would react with undeniable intensity to airborne allergens—a tingle in my nose, itching in my throat, swollen lips, and prickling sensations on my skin. In recent years, the medical narrative has shifted, acknowledging airborne allergic reactions as valid in specific situations where they've found allergenic protein particles do, in fact, become airborne.

Even so, finding reputable sources on airborne reactions remains challenging. Many articles still attribute such symptoms to anxiety and panic attacks mimicking allergic reactions rather than acknowledging legitimate airborne responses. I understand the confusion to an extent, as anxiety and allergic reactions share common symptoms. So, dismissing all airborne reactions as anxiety never felt right. As the medical field evolves, it's taught me a lesson in learning to believe in myself, my body, and what I intuitively know. I've met so many other individuals over the years who also know they are airborne allergic and have experienced similar gaslighting as me in doctor's offices and online.

Now, these once-dismissed "imaginative" reactions have been validated by research. And while I believe in science and trust it, I also recognize that the medical field is still catching up to people's lived food allergy experiences. A complaint or symptom must appear frequently enough to justify research and the subsequent approval for a study. This process is slow and deliberate, and the world of food allergies is highly nuanced. I've learned to approach the medical field with a thoughtful skepticism while also trusting my own body and experiences. I hope anyone with a new or understudied medical condition reading this feels validated.

Being repeatedly told that my airborne reactions weren't real prompted me to start documenting each close proximity peanut reaction I experienced. Whether walking through my college cafeteria, visiting a friend's office, or hanging out in a public art studio, I noticed a pattern: I remained calm when the signs suddenly began. This was a clear sign that my reactions were not anxiety-induced, as doctors had repeatedly told me they likely were.

Despite this evidence, I spent years suppressing my own understanding, convincing myself otherwise due to the confident assertions of my medical practitioners, who believed my experiences were incorrect.

It wasn't until reactions from unseen peanut particles happened again and again, like déjà vu, that I realized I was stuck in a cyclical dance of self-doubt and uncertainty. One that, not to mention, wasn't serving me in any way or getting me anywhere closer to an answer on how to stop having allergic reactions. It felt like I was constantly ping-ponging between questioning whether I was genuinely having an allergic reaction or not. After experiencing enough of these episodes in relaxed circumstances, I recognized that the validity of my experience was a tangible truth, firmly grounded in reality—not merely something "all in my mind," as I had been repeatedly told.

Realizing how much of my power I'd surrendered to the medical system, I felt a surge of frustration vibrate through me. I had entrusted my narrative to others, relinquishing control over my own story for most of my life. I wasn't giving it up any longer.

My final "aha moment," when I fully accepted that I was *positively* airborne allergic to peanuts, occurred while I was in college, interning at a local art gallery. I arrived for my shift to find the place empty; it seemed it would just be me and the gallery manager that day, who was planning to hang artwork for an upcoming show. The gallery was a sprawling converted warehouse with tall ceilings and weathered, exposed brick walls—an industrial chic vibe. The weather was pleasantly sunny in the 70s, so the front door was propped open. A cool breeze blew lightly as I strolled into the space, carefree like the air around me.

Typically, the gallery space featured little more than the art on display and a few haphazardly placed chairs or couches scattered throughout. However, that day was different.

Dozens of collapsed plastic tables lined the walls, standing upright and creating a scene reminiscent of oversized dominoes teetering on the brink of toppling. While initially alarmed by the sheer number of precariously placed white plastic tables, I continued walking to the desk area to log my arrival time.

As I walked deeper into the room, I felt a faint, bumblebee-like tingle swirling inside my nostrils—an early sign of a potential allergic reaction that I recognized all too well. I tried to dismiss it; after all, I was alone in a vast, open space with the door wide open for fresh air, and I hadn't touched or eaten anything recently. I focused on taking slow, deep breaths with long exhales to calm my nerves. I removed my jacket, placed my phone in my purse, swung it over my arm, and began searching for my intern lead.

Before I could find her, my bottom lip began getting hot and swollen. I decided to step back outside to get some fresh air, assess my next steps, and do a body scan. I opened my purse to ensure my epinephrine injectors and antihistamines were within easy reach. Confirming I did, I exited through the same open door I had entered. It occurred to me that my friend Jane had mentioned she was working a poetry event at the same gallery earlier that day. I texted her to see if they might have had peanut-containing food at the event. I was hoping to ease my mind and squash any nervousness I was having once and for all.

I fully expected a "No," a "No idea," or a delayed response.

Instead, within seconds, I received a reply in all caps: "OH MY GOD, ZOE, GET OUT OF THERE!" Then came another text: "THERE WERE PILES OF SNICKERS AT THE CENTER OF EVERY TABLE!" And another: "AND THERE WERE LIKE 40 TABLES!"

My stomach sank. I could feel myself growing pale. Dawning on me that the allergic reaction I was trying to deny was actually happening, I bolted back inside to grab my jacket and ran back out, holding my breath the entire time I was inside. Thank goodness that door was open! It made the whole process easier.

I popped two antihistamines in my mouth, took a swig from my water bottle in my car, and texted my manager at the gallery that I was having an allergic reaction, seemingly from the peanut candy consumed in the space earlier that day. I told her I was sorry about not being able to get my intern hours in, but that I'd contact her soon to reschedule.

As I drove home, I called my mom on speaker to let her know what was happening, but I made it clear that I thought I'd be okay since it was an airborne exposure only. She made me promise to continue monitoring my symptoms and not hesitate to administer my epinephrine injector and call 911 if need be.

After this happened, no argument could convince me otherwise: reacting to airborne food particles was possible. It may be considered "rare," but I was all too familiar with receiving that label in the medical field.

I often felt like a medical curiosity in the eyes of physicians. I've lost count of how many times doctors have told me, "This is unusual and not the norm." But this supposed rarity is an illusion—it's a real trend that no one is documenting or taking seriously. I've seen this pattern repeatedly in both the food allergy and autoimmune communities. I can only imagine how many others experience the same thing: when something falls outside the currently understood "norm," it's often dismissed as rare or impossible.

This isn't just frustrating, it's isolating. It creates a dynamic where your lived experience is treated as an anomaly, a one-off, a fluke. But what if it's common? What if it's simply not yet understood because no one is taking it seriously and it is not being tracked?

It's disheartening to realize how widespread this kind of dismissal is—not just in medicine, but across the psychological fields and beyond. And to think about how long it's been happening: centuries. Living with my peanut allergy has taught me not to discredit what others say about their own bodies. I trust people when they describe their symptoms. For me, it's about trusting the scientific evidence while also recognizing that our understanding isn't fixed. It can be incomplete, sometimes under-researched, and always subject to change as we learn more. I've seen this firsthand with food allergy medical advice, which has swung sometimes a full 180 degrees over the past few decades.

I was told my diagnosis of autoimmune psoriatic arthritis (PsA) was practically unheard of in young women, yet within the past few years of my diagnosis I have met at least five other women in my own community, all diagnosed in their 20s and 30s. The raised eyebrows, the hesitations, the implicit questions: *Are you sure? Could it be anxiety? This isn't common in women, though.* It's as though the burden of proof lies entirely on those of us living with these conditions.

But here's the thing: the more stories I hear like this from others, the clearer it becomes that while the medical field knows a lot, there is still so much more we don't fully understand. After COVID-19, I began to see more and more in people around me how our immune systems can react to stressors in complex ways, how an infection or stressful experience can set off new immune-related conditions, and flares that trigger or worsen existing ones.

The Cleveland Clinic explains that if you have an autoimmune disease, your immune system is more active than it should be, and when there aren't invaders to attack, it can turn on your body and damage healthy tissue. The NIH notes that autoimmune disorders occur with increased frequency in patients who already have another autoimmune disease, estimating that about 25 percent of patients with an autoimmune disease will develop additional autoimmune disorders.

We know that women, especially women of color, have been historically excluded from clinical studies—or, in some cases, studied without consent, particularly among marginalized populations. Looking closely at sample sizes for studies and research populations has been eye-opening. Maybe something is "not common" in someone like me simply because it hasn't been studied *in* someone like me. Or maybe there's never been funding for it in the first place—especially when it comes to women's health. For decades, medical research routinely excluded women, treating our bodies as outliers instead of the norm, and we're still living with the consequences of that deliberate exclusion.

This disbelief is more than just inconvenient, though; it's dangerous. When our realities are minimized or dismissed, it leads to misdiagnosis, delayed treatments, and an overall lack of resources and support. It perpetuates the myth that specific reactions or conditions "hardly ever happen" when they happen far more often than anyone realizes. This skepticism can seep into how we view ourselves. We begin questioning our own experiences, minimizing our struggles because the world around us seems unwilling to validate them.

Food allergies and their many nuances are not easy to define. They're messy, layered, and varied. By brushing off anything beyond the standard narrative, we risk, as a society, leaving countless people in the shadows, unheard and unprotected. It's not about being believed for the sake of validation—it's about ensuring safety, understanding, and progress. Until more people in the medical field start putting the patient first and listening, we'll all continue to mistake the misunderstood for the nonexistent.

Thankfully, I'd recently read the book *The Invisible Kingdom* by Meghan O'Rourke, which fully validated my many experiences of being doubted by those in the medical field. Her vulnerable book shares insight into her experiences of being told her symptoms were in her head: spoiler alert, they weren't. It makes me think about how many others in the food allergy community believe they're airborne, yet have been made to feel foolish for saying so. My question is: why and how would hundreds of people who don't know one another make this up? *The Invisible Kingdom* illuminates that simply because symptoms are understudied, misunderstood, and not researched, doesn't mean they're all in our minds.

After numerous similar reactions in unmistakable clarity, I was done holding out hope and pretending I wasn't airborne allergic. No more placating doctors. Inside me, there was an understandable desire and internal temptation to embrace the comforting notion that it wasn't possible to react this way, which undoubtedly would have rendered my life more straightforward, and less fear ridden.

Cross-Contact

In high school, my best friend turned me on to the simple joy of unwrapping individual Dove chocolates, appreciating their cute, uplifting messages on the wrapper while savoring their silky-smooth chocolate. It was like a little fortune cookie but with decadent chocolate instead. Every so often, I'd buy a bag at the grocery store and keep it in the fridge because I especially love eating chocolate cold.

One evening at home, I wandered into the kitchen and reached into my bag of chocolates. A twinge of disappointment hit me as I realized I was down to just two—I usually enjoyed them four at a time. Determined to savor my last treats, I carried them to my bedroom, settled in at my computer, and started streaming a TV show.

When I unwrapped one and popped it into my mouth, a peanut-like smell hit me immediately, followed by a metallic taste. I spit it out as quickly as I could, but it was hard to remove. I had already bitten into it with my front teeth and started swirling a small piece around, melting the chocolate with my tongue.

I dashed into the bathroom, brushing my mouth out with my toothbrush, making a mental note that it would need to be discarded later. I could feel my lip swelling, and the poisonous taste was unmistakable. After making sure my mouth was reasonably cleaned out, I texted my roommates to alert them of the situation and took two antihistamines.

Over the next several minutes, I kept taking more antihistamine medicine to control the reaction, but I could feel it worsening instead of improving. Before I knew it, I had taken around eight or nine pills. At that point in my life, this was my protocol: I would monitor myself closely and only stop taking antihistamines once I felt the reaction had stopped escalating. I was afraid to use the epinephrine and didn't understand when it was appropriate to do so.

I learned from experience that taking this much antihistamine, which typically makes people sleepy and drowsy, can also have the opposite effect and make you hyper. Additionally, I've come to understand that there are more serious consequences at play with this method, as only epinephrine will stop anaphylaxis.

So there I was, jittery and wide awake at 10pm with an early work morning ahead of me, dealing with the aftermath of the reaction I finally felt I had under control. I curled into the large, comfy chair in my room, clutching my phone in case I needed to call someone. Tears spilled out of me, trying to be kind to myself, but the disappointment in not using my epinephrine cut deep. I knew this wasn't sustainable—that my fear of the needle jamming into my intramuscular thigh could one day cost me everything, especially if I was alone when the reaction hit.

For a long time I treated my epinephrine injector as a last resort, when really it's the immediate, life-saving step. I'm practicing the affirmation provided by Thomas Silvera of the Elijah-Alavi Foundation: "Don't fear the device, fear the delay." This is why epinephrine alternatives to the needle feel so revolutionary to me, and why I'm grateful non-needle options like nasal sprays are finally here. This story happened many years before the allergy community widely understood the urgency of the now-common saying, "Epi first, Epi fast," and that antihistamines shouldn't be taken in such large quantities for multiple reasons such as side effects and even potential overdose. It wasn't until my late twenties that I grasped how antihistamine medications, while helpful, could actually mask the critical signs of anaphylaxis, potentially delaying the crucial use of epinephrine, which is ultimately the sole life-saving treatment.

The next day, I started questioning how I'd safely eaten from the same bag of chocolates, only to react to a random chocolate at the bottom of the bag. This was before the social media era we know today, around 2013, when food allergies and labeling laws weren't as commonly discussed. I wasn't yet aware of the term "cross-contact," and this incident made me wonder if peanuts were in the same facility as these chocolates. The chocolates didn't list peanuts in the ingredients panel, but I wondered if they could have contained trace amounts, as the taste of peanuts was unmistakable.

After this chocolate incident, I spent the next week going down an absolute rabbit hole trying to find out if products "may contain" my allergens in an undisclosed way. I learned that labeling around "may contain" and "trace amounts" in the US was voluntary and not regulated, the same way it is today. I also discovered that only the top allergens are required to be labeled if they're purposefully in a product. This began my era of reaching out to companies before I ate a food product, which is still how I manage my food allergy today due to the lack of labeling law protections.

Reaching out to every food brand and inquiring about

allergens in the facility was, and still can be, extremely time-consuming. When I first started, it led to many disappointing email replies and a lack of responses. But doing this felt necessary to get a handle on my reactions. It was a frustrating yet exciting time in my life.

Once I stopped eating products from facilities that used my anaphylactic allergen, peanut, my allergic reactions significantly decreased. Because of this, I wanted to shout from the rooftops about our lack of transparency in labeling in the United States. *How did I just learn about this,* I thought, *in my twenties!* Before I cut these potentially contaminated products out, I had reactions almost weekly, if not more, and was living in a constant state of confusion and fear around managing my allergy.

While I still maintain a healthy level of caution regarding food allergy fears, it no longer controls my life as it once did. This newfound understanding of the dangers of food labeling inspired me to start my blog, *Invisibly Allergic*, in 2017. I aimed to share what helped me uncover the root of my reactions—cross-contact from trace amounts of my allergen on shared equipment or within shared food manufacturing facilities.

Suddenly, I felt empowered to share my story, and the blogging process was therapeutic in many ways. If only a handful of people visited my website, it would be a success. Fast forward to present day: with no paid advertisements, my site now receives thousands of views and visits each month. I offer free resources and free consultations, as my site is driven solely by my passion for raising awareness and my desire to contribute to the transparent labeling law changes I wish to see.

Airline Travel

For those with food allergies, flying often means confronting a persistent fear of potential allergic reactions in an environment where our control is limited. Imagine being trapped in a crowded space, surrounded by surfaces that are likely coated with poison. To make matters worse, some airlines distribute this poison to everyone on board. It's scary, right?

All airlines pose the risk of someone in close proximity bringing allergens onboard for themselves, directly contaminating your space. This is the reality for 33 million others and me, not including their friends and family with whom they are likely traveling with. Despite some hard-fought wins by the allergy community leading to legal improvements in airline practices over the years, it's important to recognize that US airlines are not required to follow the same ADA guidelines we rely on in other areas of life. Additionally, food served on airlines does not have to comply with the FDA labeling standards that apply on the ground. The FDA only merely suggests accurate labeling for in-flight food, so if you have a food allergy, it's simply not worth the risk to eat airline meals.

In the US, we're used to the ADA mandating reasonable accommodations in workplaces, events, schools, and businesses. However, airlines are exempt from these rules and instead follow separate disability guidelines under the Air Carrier Access Act (ACAA). This difference is one reason discrimination on airlines is so frequently reported, affecting not only people with food allergies but also wheelchair users and others with disabilities. Organizations like All Wheels Up exist to advocate for basic wheelchair accommodations on flights—a need so critical that their work highlights the scale of the ongoing problem.

I first learned about how the ADA doesn't apply in the air from the blog The No Nut Traveler, now a non-profit. Lianne, the powerhouse behind it, started her website to collect statements of airline experiences and examine the legal aspects. Thanks to Lianne with No Nut Traveler, preboarding is now a legal requirement due to the Air Access Act. Plus, her testimonies led to the collection of significant data around reactions during flight. Not only has someone had first-time allergic reactions to food on air, but in her testimonies, it's happened more than once.

Plus, to make it worse for everyone, most flight attendants often don't want to do CPR, deliver a baby, or use an epinephrine auto-injector or syringe on someone because it's all out of their training scope and skillset. As Lianne has made clear on her website, the whole airline system must enter the 21st century and acknowledge and properly train staff on the many possibilities they could face.

Airlines have the right to kick anyone off a plane they want; ultimately, the pilot makes the call. Furthermore, you can't sue an airline; only file a DFT complaint. Lianne proves that we have to share our stories, words, and experiences, which are important and matter. We need documentation to make changes.

If you see people you follow online asking for food allergy experience surveys or any survey close to your values and heart, as long as it's not spammy and is legitimate with a clear end goal, take the time to fill those out. It's important data that is hard to get. Unfortunately, I have encountered multiple bad airline experiences, but one still haunts me the most. And I did report it to Lianne after it occurred. Spoiler alert: I got my flight reimbursed after this incident, which I'm about to describe, but this shows that a monetary refund doesn't erase the memory or the emotional impact.

It was 2011, and I was flying Southwest Airlines to New York City to visit a childhood friend. Before booking the flight, I followed my usual peanut allergy routine, which has since evolved. At the time, this meant calling the airline to inform them of my allergy and ensuring they would substitute the usual snacks for something without peanuts on my flight.

While peanuts were still served on flights before and after mine, they wouldn't be provided to guests on my specific one. I preferred booking my flights over the phone to ensure they noted my allergy in their system. At that time, Southwest, like most airlines, served peanuts as a standard "courtesy" snack. They typically accommodated my request to switch snacks without too much hassle, although some airlines flatly refused. Because of this, I only flew with the companies that would accommodate this snack switch.

In 2025, most airlines still sell snacks with top allergens, but they don't all pass them out as regularly as they used to. The early 2010s marked a time when airlines grappled with the need to switch due to food allergies. I had trouble keeping track of which airlines served peanuts and which didn't. Many would stop serving them, only to start again later. I'd send them a thank-you email to show my support when airlines stopped serving peanuts. Then, a few months later, I'd find myself emailing them again to let them know I could no longer fly with them due to a change in their policy. It was (and still is) a mess.

When I fly, I always ask to preboard so I can wipe down my seat, seatbelt, and surrounding area, and put on a KN95 mask. I tend to do this whenever I go to places where my allergens are present, like movie theaters or public venues, but the difference is that on the ground, I'm much closer to a hospital and medical care if I need it.

Preboarding also gives me a chance to tell the attendants, "I have a peanut allergy disability, my seat number is ___, and my epinephrine is in my purse." I usually try to fit in, "Would you mind making an announcement to others to refrain from eating peanut products on the flight?" too. There is a slim chance they will announce it, but I try my luck and see. It's up to the individual flight attendants to decide, so it's often not something they will do in advance.

On this particular flight to NYC, I sat in my freshly wiped, damp seat and watched people filling in around me. The flight crew announced to the fully boarded plane that this was a peanut-free flight and no peanuts would be served. They also asked anyone bringing peanut products to refrain from eating them. I was elated! A smile spread beneath my KN95 mask, the edges pinching the corners of my eyes. A considerable weight melted off my shoulders. That's when I heard the man behind me push the call button for the flight attendant. My gut told me he was about to comment on the peanut announcement.

"Excuse me, I brought peanuts on board; can I just eat them anyway?" the man asked. "Yeah, you can eat them; we just say that, but it doesn't actually mean anything," the flight attendant replied.

My eyes widened in disbelief. *Doesn't actually mean anything? Then why say it?* I thought to myself. As she walked away, I turned to face the strawberry-blonde-haired man behind me, still wearing his sunglasses and looking no older than 40.

He said abruptly before I could even say anything, "I had a feeling I was sitting near the person with the peanut allergy." "Yep, that's me!" I replied, trying to stay calm and appear more relaxed than I felt. I followed up with, "I asked them to make that announcement because I'm airborne allergic to peanuts and could have a potential reaction. If that happened, it could delay the entire plane with an emergency landing. So that's why they said it." He just looked at me, so I continued, "I'm surprised she said the announcement didn't mean anything because they offered it to me as an accommodation. Unfortunately, I can react if you eat peanuts this close to me." I said through my mask.

We talked back and forth for the next 5 minutes as I strained my neck over my seat. He was initially stern with many questions, but as I answered, he softened. He eventually explained that his son has a friend on his soccer team with a peanut allergy who is the same as me and can't be around peanut products. He said because of that, he "gets it." I questioned that, especially after his rapid-fire interrogation. But whatever. I found myself divulging a lot of personal information, justifying why my life is more important than this specific food to a stranger—ultimately, none of his business. However, when I successfully change someone's perspective, I feel like a *badass*—not going to lie.

That day, the conversation worked in my favor. I thanked him for not eating the peanuts he brought and offered him one of my extra snacks if he would like it. He declined, and I turned around in my seat. I firmly pressed my mask against my nose and continued the flight, knowing everyone around us heard our public discussion. I hoped it helped ensure no one else nearby ate peanuts.

At that moment, I made a plan to call Southwest Airlines after my flight to let them know what their attendant said in their announcement. I understand they can't guarantee that no one on the flight will eat my allergen, but to say "it doesn't mean anything" right after making the announcement was inappropriate. A more accurate statement would have been, "Someone nearby has a life-threatening peanut allergy, so we're asking people to refrain," which would have been much preferred.

After discussing the incident with the airline over the phone, they reimbursed my flight—a genuinely nice gesture and the only time that's happened to me. I suggested they implement allergy training for flight attendants. I thanked the crew members on board who made the initial allergy announcement, as it was not the same woman who spoke to the passenger behind me.

Fast forward to July 2024, I found myself again navigating the complexities of flying with a peanut allergy, this time on an Allegiant Airlines flight. As I pre-boarded, I approached the flight attendants to inform them of my life-threatening peanut allergy, my seat number, and the location of my epinephrine in my bag. I also asked if they could make an announcement requesting passengers to refrain from eating peanuts. However, they informed me that they couldn't comply due to onboard sales of peanut M&Ms. I already knew this from their website, but I hoped that, perhaps, I'd get lucky and they would choose to make an announcement after all.

As I turned to walk to my seat, the pilot, who was standing with the attendants, called out to me, "I'll make sure we pass out complimentary peanuts to your aisle—haha." I was baffled and responded with a simple "Oh no… I hope not" before continuing to my seat.

That's when my friend, preboarding with me, remarked within earshot of the pilot, "Wow, Zoë, that's frustrating. What makes people say things like this to you?" I didn't have an immediate response, but once we reached our seats, I told her, "I have no idea—maybe ignorance. You'd think an airline pilot would be aware of the incidents involving allergies on planes, including deaths and emergency landings." Feeling drained, I settled into my seat and secured my mask.

A few minutes later, after overhearing the pilot's remark, a flight attendant approached me with a generous handful of wet wipes. She shared that her son also has a peanut allergy similar to mine and advised me to wipe down my area thoroughly, saying, "You never know what someone ate here earlier." Her gesture of kindness spoke volumes, and we exchanged a knowing look, silently acknowledging the pilot's insensitivity.

Navigating food allergies while flying can be a minefield, which is why resources like Lianne's are so valuable. Another incredible resource is Laurel Francouer, a writer and attorney who specializes in food allergy law and policy. Through her website, allergylawyer.com, Laurel provides expert legal guidance for those dealing with allergies in many settings, including air travel.

You may know her from the widely publicized Panera case, where she represented a family who were served a grilled cheese sandwich with peanut butter dollop on it after telling the Panera staff their daughter was peanut-allergic. I appreciate how Laurel has always highlighted how our current laws have not kept pace with the needs of the allergy community. In addition to her legal work, Laurel co-authored the *Preschool Allergy Handbook* with Gina Minnett Lee, M.Ed, providing best practices to help keep young children safe in school settings.

Through Laurel, I also learned about advocacy organizations like COPASA—Councils of Parent Attorneys and Advocates—who provide great resources and community support on platforms like Instagram and Facebook, helping families navigate the complex legal landscape around food allergies.

Closing Thoughts & Additional Context

- Epi First, Epi Fast: Epinephrine is a life-saving drug, but its effectiveness depends on several factors and is not guaranteed. According to a 2023 National Institutes of Health article, "Injectable epinephrine is the first-line treatment for anaphylaxis. Epinephrine is touted as 'life-saving,' particularly because observational studies have identified the lack of prompt epinephrine treatment as a critical risk factor associated with anaphylaxis fatality." This highlights the urgency behind the common saying "Epi first, Epi fast"—because it truly can save a life. If you have a needle phobia, there are many strategies to help manage it while still carrying your life-saving medication. Plus, there is a needle-free option called Neffy, a nasal spray version of epinephrine. There's also Aquestive's dissolvable epinephrine product, Anaphylm, a sublingual film designed to treat allergic reactions like anaphylaxis by dissolving under the tongue for rapid epinephrine delivery. It's currently on track for FDA approval, so keep an eye out for this promising new option. If you suspect anaphylaxis, use any form of epinephrine. There are no downsides to epinephrine, and any pain will be forgotten in the grand scheme, I promise. Take it from someone who hates needles—the fear is always worse than the shot itself, and epinephrine can save your life.

- Limitations of Antihistamines: No antihistamine can reverse anaphylaxis—you need epinephrine for that. In fact, antihistamines can sometimes mask the symptoms of anaphylaxis, delaying the use of epinephrine when it's urgently needed. While antihistamines can help alleviate allergy symptoms, they work too slowly to manage a life-threatening reaction. According to the Mayo Clinic, epinephrine is the only treatment for anaphylaxis. In February 2024, the FDA approved Xolair for food allergies to help reduce the severity of allergic reactions. If interested, ask your allergist to learn more about this potential therapeutic option. I've started Xolair myself and am eager to see whether it reduces my reactivity, particularly to airborne triggers. Now over 20 weeks into treatment, I'm observing whether it alters the frequency or intensity of my reactions. The food allergy field is still, in many ways, in its infancy, so it will be interesting to see how allergy management continues to evolve. Depending on the individual, different treatments may be recommended. But as more options become available, it can also become more confusing—especially when general awareness around these treatments isn't widely shared or accessible.

- Airline Disability Guidelines: Airlines do not follow the same ADA guidelines we are familiar with in the US. "Discrimination by air carriers in areas other than employment is not covered by the ADA but rather by the Air Carrier Access Act (49 U.S.C. 1374 (c))," explained by the ADA National Network.

- Airline Statistics on Food Allergy Reactions: A CFAAR study taken between October 2022 and November 2022 showed the challenges families with food allergies face in air travel. A Healio article found, "A survey of 4,704 people affected by food allergy revealed 400 in-flight incidents, including five cases requiring an emergency landing."

- US Cross-Contact and Labeling Issues: Cross-contact and "may contain" labeling leave much to be desired for those who depend on this information for life-threatening food allergens. Only the top 9 allergens must be labeled if they are purposefully in a product. This includes ingredients derived from a top 9 allergen if they contain protein from that allergen, but highly refined or processed forms that do not contain the allergenic protein are not required to be labeled, even if they're from a top 9 allergen. They are also not required to be listed if present accidentally or in trace amounts due to equipment and processing. Even then, recalls happen when the ingredient label information is incorrect. I need to know what allergens are in the facility to make an informed choice about eating the product. I also highly recommend reading about and signing the petition by SnackSafely on Change.org, titled *Urgent Call to FDA: Reform Dangerous Food Allergy Labeling Ambiguity NOW!*

- Airborne Reactions Are Real and Valid: A 2009 National Institute of Health (NIH) research article stated on airborne reactions: "Though not widely recognized, food hypersensitivity by inhalation can cause major morbidity in affected individuals. The exposure is usually more obvious and often substantial in occupational environments but frequently occurs in non-occupational settings, such as homes, schools, restaurants, grocery stores, and commercial flights. The exposure can be trivial, as in mere smelling or being in the vicinity of the food. The clinical manifestations can vary from a benign respiratory or cutaneous reaction to a systemic one that can be life-threatening. In addition to strict avoidance, such highly sensitive subjects should carry epinephrine and wear MedicAlert identification." I imagine airborne allergies will be much more frequently discussed as a valid part of the food allergy experience in the next decade.

4

ANAPHYLAXIS AT THE ALLERGIST

May 23, 2013

This chapter recounts the first and only time that I experienced anaphylactic shock leading to a complete loss of consciousness. Even after more than a decade, reflecting on the turn of events still leaves me baffled. I'll never forget the moment I regained my vision, staring at my reflection in the mirror, barely recognizing myself. My face, neck, and extremities were painted in a hauntingly deep purple-blue hue, a sign of oxygen deprivation.

The truth is, I nearly died while under medical care, all in response to what I was told was routine allergy testing. Before this occurred, I was misled to believe anaphylaxis was not likely. I'm sharing my anaphylactic story in hopes that it helps others stay strong when advocating for themselves to medical staff regarding their food allergies. I feel it's particularly important to raise awareness about the possibility of false negatives during allergy scratch and prick tests or any test that involves contact with your known allergens.

I'm sharing this not to provoke fear, but to encourage everyone to talk with their allergist before undergoing any intradermal skin allergy testing, especially for potential or known life-threatening allergens. I recently spoke with a board-certified allergist who said intradermal testing for food is an outdated practice that should rarely be used, particularly for known allergens, because of the high risk of anaphylaxis. Since the story I'm about to recount happened a decade ago, I hope no doctors are still using this outdated method, which is no longer recommended for testing allergens.

If my story can help even one person avoid what I went

through during a standard initial consultation, I've done what I've set out to do here. As you'll learn from this story and may already know from your own experiences, not all allergist offices are created equal, and not all operate with the best interest of their patients in mind.

A version of this first appeared on *Invisibly Allergic* in 2017. It featured a high-contrast image of an emergency room door—fitting because you'd think that's where I would have ended up after going into anaphylaxis. However, things didn't go as expected; I was not taken to a hospital. Despite the clear protocol on epinephrine packaging at the time, which advised monitoring in an ER after an anaphylactic reaction, I was instructed to drive myself home from the most highly rated allergist's office in my city, just hours after regaining consciousness.

Medical care after anaphylactic shock is suggested because it involves monitoring changes in breathing, oxygen levels, and the potential for a biphasic reaction, where a second anaphylactic response occurs without re-exposure to the allergen. Looking back, I'm grateful I made it home safely, as I was completely lethargic and drowsy.

It was April 2013, and I'd reached my breaking point with recurring allergic reactions to foods that didn't list peanut ingredients—my deadly allergen. Frustrated, I visited my primary care doctor, eager to see an allergist who could help me manage these unpredictable reactions. I wondered if allergy shots might lessen my sensitivity to environmental allergies and, possibly, help control my reactions to peanuts. My doctor referred me to the most reputable allergist in town, and I promptly made an appointment.

When I called and spoke to the allergist's office, they were surprised I had never undergone a full allergy testing panel and felt they could help me get some answers if I agreed to various allergy panels. At age 23, I was told I would undergo a prick test to check for allergies tied to my asthma and to identify all my allergens, including food allergies. After the tests were completed, we would discuss the results.

I could've sworn I had mentioned my upcoming appointment to my mom, but afterward, she told me she would have advised against a prick test and suggested I only do blood work especially if I was alone. She always believed that exposing me directly to potential allergens—especially to peanuts—was too risky. In hindsight, her advice is glaringly clear, and thinking back on what I could've avoided makes me recoil.

When scheduling the appointment, I knew my mom would offer to come with me if I wanted, but as a young adult craving independence, I felt a strong urge to face this alone. I wanted to identify my allergic reactions and share the results with her afterward. I was determined to handle the testing on my own, not wanting anyone to take time off work on my account. But I never anticipated the visit would take such a dangerous turn. I've often wondered how differently that day might have gone if I'd brought someone along—someone who could help advocate for me and support me as I advocated for myself.

In 2013, online food allergy communities were less developed than now, and food allergy educational resources were more challenging to find. Back then, if I had to describe my food allergy, I would have said, "My allergic reactions are out of control, with no rhyme or reason." This horrible anaphylaxis episode at the allergist's office was a turning point for me, as it motivated me to educate myself about food allergies and uncover the concept of cross-contact to trace amounts of my allergen. Ultimately, through my research, my reactions were very predictable and almost always triggered by trace amounts of peanuts that were undeclared in the foods I consumed.

Due to the US's lack of comprehensive FDA food labeling laws, food manufacturers aren't required to disclose potential undeclared allergens that may transfer onto products. As of the publication of this book, the FDA's requirements are limited to declaring allergens only if a product intentionally contains the top 9 allergens. There are no regulations or consequences for "may contain" or precautionary labeling statements, nor are there any requirements regarding allergens present due to shared equipment or facilities. I've found that many people, whether impacted by food allergies or not, are surprised by this. I explain more about how to decode food labels in Chapter 6.

Something else worth noting, which I touched on before, is that if the top allergens required to be labeled are "refined oils," they are exempt from FDA labeling. So, if ice cream contains refined peanut oil, it does not need to be labeled as "contains: peanuts." This seems particularly ridiculous to me. I have followed this advice and eaten potato chips fried in peanut oil and reacted to it. While my reaction was not anaphylaxis, I did need antihistamines, and it was frightening as I monitored whether it would progress. After this, I researched and learned that refining processes vary widely and are not all equal, so there could still be proteins present. Why risk it?

Equally alarming, companies can legally label products as "nut-free" or "allergy-friendly" without these claims being accurate, defined, or regulated. This lack of transparency and the risk of cross-contact in food manufacturing has become my primary focus for change within the food industry. My goal is to prevent life-threatening reactions and improve the mental well-being of those managing food allergies. I also aim to advance food allergy awareness by sharing my experience and uplifting others in the space.

Regarding food labeling laws, providing clear, transparent ingredient information to the public is essential for enabling everyone—regardless of whether they have food allergies—to make informed choices about what they consume. Everyone deserves the right to make educated and informed decisions about what they're eating, whether due to food allergies, intolerances, dietary restrictions, or personal preferences.

This lack of transparency is deeply frustrating, especially knowing that food manufacturers could take steps to access the information consumers need about what's in their facilities. That knowledge could significantly improve the lives of millions of families. If they don't already have this information readily available, they absolutely should find it out. After all, they are running businesses meant to provide people with safe food. With at least 33 million people in the US and their families relying on accurate labeling, this information must be disclosed. Unfortunately, that's not the case right now, so we need to push for policies that address this common-sense, non-partisan issue.

In January 2025, the US Food and Drug Administration (FDA) updated its allergen labeling guidance, reclassifying coconut as a fruit rather than a tree nut and removing the requirement for it to be labeled as a major allergen on packaged foods. It was an update to the Food Allergen Labeling and Consumer Protection Act (FALCPA) reclassifying coconut. However, instead of simply redefining it, regulators removed the requirement for coconut to be labeled as a major allergen on packaged foods.

This change was a significant setback for the food allergy community, as many individuals are severely allergic to coconut. In addition, other ingredients with "nut" in the name—such as shea nut, which are actually seeds—were also excluded from allergen labeling requirements. These ingredients were already being labeled before, so removing them offered no added benefit and introduced serious risks. The change was not widely publicized, leaving many in the community unaware, which is especially dangerous for those with coconut allergies. To make matters more confusing, when you search online to see if coconut is considered a tree nut, many AI-generated answers still reflect outdated information—stating it must be labeled under current food allergen labeling laws, which is no longer true. The lack of transparency and disregard for allergic individuals has left many feeling frustrated, confused, and at greater risk.

I thrive on moving actions forward, tackling challenges, and embracing a mindset of figuring things out even when unsure of the exact path ahead. Recently, I discussed this aspect of my personality with my therapist. While I haven't pinpointed exactly where this drive comes from, we've identified that I've been an activist since I was a preteen—something I've never truly acknowledged or given much thought to before.

By age 11, I organized my first protest in coordination with People for the Ethical Treatment of Animals (PETA) against a new Kentucky Fried Chicken location being built at the end of my street. Although the restaurant ultimately opened, I felt deep satisfaction from fighting for a cause I believed in. I was comforted by the collective awareness I raised and the sense of care and community that came out of the protest.

I've advocated for human and animal rights from an early age, especially considering my lifelong vegetarianism. I often reflect on how much safer life could be for everyone, particularly for low-income individuals like myself growing up, who may need help understanding the risks posed by gaps in our food labeling laws. Lacking access to allergists or education about these critical issues leaves them the most vulnerable. Observing these disparities and recognizing the higher rates of food allergies in low-income and marginalized communities drives me to work toward creating equity in the food allergy and disability spaces, among others.

When discussing medical experiences and my qualifications in the food allergy space, I strive to be forthright about the limits of my knowledge. I have no formal education on intradermal allergy testing; everything I know is based on my personal experiences, conversations with others, and online research. Based on my allergy paperwork, the day I went into anaphylaxis at the allergist's office

I was tested for 76 different allergens through skin-prick testing on my back, where droplets of allergen were placed on the skin and lightly pricked, and intradermal testing on my arms, where a small amount of allergen was injected just under the skin.

Before I get into the rest of the unsettling details, I have to pause and say—this part of the testing was excruciating. I'm not exaggerating when I say I was literally dripping blood from the tests. The needles sharply pierced my skin far deeper than I had imagined. Concerned that the person administering the test wasn't doing it correctly because of the pain, I couldn't help but ask—as politely as possible—if it was supposed to hurt that much. I held back tears as I watched the needles sink into my skin.

My bloody arms tensed in pain, and as I looked down at the purple and black marker patterns covering my upper body, I felt like a human dry-erase board—an experience I was mentally unprepared for that day, to say the least. I remember thinking, *what am I doing here? How did I end up in this situation?*

Getting Tested

At the start of my appointment, I made one thing crystal clear: I told the allergist I didn't need to be tested for peanuts. I was already certain of my life-long allergy and carried both EpiPens and antihistamines. I could read on their faces that they wanted to test me for it anyway and were skeptical, wanting to rely on their tests instead of my word.

Because of this, I confidently told them I was so allergic that if they brought peanut butter into the room and ate it, I would start showing symptoms like a swollen lip. I knew this because it had recently happened, so I hoped sharing it would reassure them.

They wanted to test me for peanuts anyway, saying that I may not be allergic to the nut itself and that it could be the fungus that grows on them instead and explained that they needed to find out. I let them know I was uncomfortable with it, and they assured me it was safe and advantageous that I be tested for peanuts since I had never had formal allergy testing done for my allergy. In the end, I advocated for myself as best I could at that moment. Still, eventually, I was talked into being tested for peanuts by a few doctors and/or nurses there, saying it was routine and expected to be tested for your known allergen(s).

I was so incredibly nervous with the idea of the test that I began to feel flustered, sweating, and panicky. Multiple nurses and doctors came in to address my distress, each explaining that they wanted to perform a prick test specifically on the underside of my forearm for peanuts to differentiate it from the rest of my testing. However, their explanations only made me more concerned, as I repeatedly insisted that I didn't need to be tested for peanuts and wasn't feeling heard.

To this day, I don't know why I didn't walk out of the allergist's office right then and there. I felt I didn't have the choice to say no, even though I absolutely did. In fact, I did say no multiple times, but they continued to not take my *no* as an answer. Feeling worn down, I reluctantly went along with their plan, trusting their team's expertise over my own understanding of my peanut allergy. Regrettably, I allowed the peanut testing to be done on my arm.

Minutes later, they told me I wasn't allergic to peanuts.

"Excuse me, what?" I said. "Sorry, but that can't be right, I've been allergic to peanuts my whole life." So, they showed me, tilting the underside of my forearm up towards my face with a prideful *I told you so* expression.

They let me know I was not allergic to peanuts in a very matter-of-fact way, pointing to my pale arm with no noticeable reaction. They laughed and said, "I know it's confusing, but it's true. You aren't allergic to peanuts, so it must be something else. This is good news!"

While this made no sense to me, I saw it with my own eyes—

my arm showed no evidence of a reaction. Meanwhile, other areas of my body definitely showed reactions to the other 70+ allergens I was being tested for. They proceeded to let me know I was highly allergic to cockroaches, dust mites, birch trees, oak trees, mold, ragweed, grass, and other environmental allergens based on the large welts on my back and arms.

However, I wouldn't let them breeze past this new information about peanuts because I knew it was incorrect. I explained that I am baffled, but that their test is not right. They assured me the test was correct and said to be sure, they wanted to test me a second time for peanuts in the same area of my arm. As wooziness rippled throughout my body, I chalked it up to being stuck by a ton of needles, feeling uneasy with the situation, and being in a medium amount of physical pain.

I was in a state of shock. Being told I wasn't allergic to peanuts when I knew I was. They flipped over my arm and proceeded to test my same arm a second time, this time closer to my wrist, to prove I wasn't allergic. Then exited the room and closed the door behind them, leaving me, for a second time, by myself. There were still no visible signs of a reaction on my arm, and there never was any sign of a reaction on my arm.

In an attempt to distract myself, I turned to social media. I picked up my phone and posted a bewildered Facebook status: "I'm apparently not allergic to peanuts, but maybe to the fungus on them or something else???" I began snapping pictures of my arms and back with my cell phone, getting a better view of the purple and black markings—a visual summary of the day's bizarre turn. Behind me, a cute but out-of-place puppy poster stared down at me from the wall.

Suddenly I was overcome by a creeping, warm, tingling sensation moving up my spine. I started getting dizzy and lightheaded. The last thing I remember is walking out of the room into the hall, calling for a nurse to help me because my vision was going out, and I was sweating profusely, feeling faint and hot. I knew what was happening. She knew what was happening. The edges of my vision closed in until there was nothing—just black.

I had the scary realization that I couldn't find my purse with my epinephrine. Even though I was adamant about always carrying them, I didn't even know what direction I was standing. It was my worst fear, and I was going into anaphylaxis from these nonsensical peanut skin pricks I didn't want in the first place. I began lowering myself to the ground, leaning my body weight into the wall behind me until I collapsed.

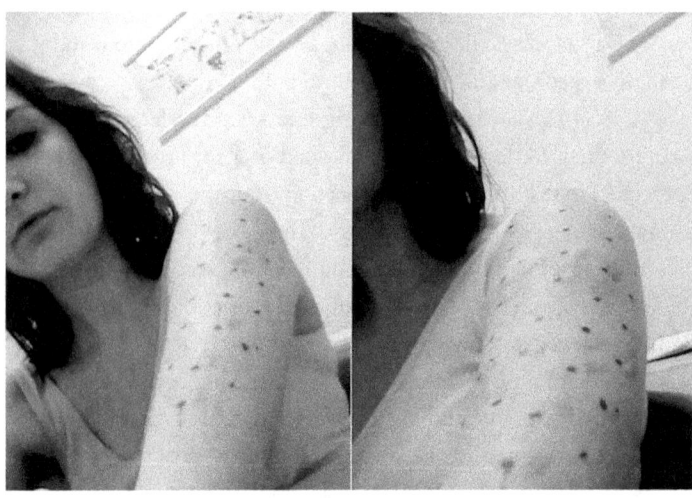

At the allergist's office, moments before my unexpected anaphylactic reaction—May 23, 2013.

The Throes of Anaphylaxis

It was pitch black. I had the sensation that I was floating in the vast emptiness of space, cut off from everything. My hearing vanished entirely, replaced by a squeezing sensation in my ears—like the pressure that builds when you're driving through mountains and your ears need to pop. Everything was eerily silent. A sense of nothingness washed over me, and I realized I couldn't hear my heartbeat or pulse. I couldn't even feel myself breathing.

The familiar weight of my body and extremities vanished, revealing a sensation I usually took for granted. In its place was an overwhelming sense of light that felt alien and disorienting. I began to think I was dying and made peace with it. As if watching myself on a movie screen, I floated away into a dark abyss, watching my body drift further into the distance. I experienced zero discomfort, no pain or agony, only complete calm.

To this day, I'm unsure exactly how long I was unconscious—my best guess is between 2 to 4 minutes. They had administered three epinephrine injectors and a steroid shot, and I started to see flashes of light from the ceiling above and managed to blink my heavy eyelids open with just a faint crack. Though I couldn't hear anything, I could tell I was slowly coming back.

The sensation of returning to life is almost indescribable. I gradually became more and more aware of my surroundings. Panic set in as I noticed my discolored purple-gray limbs looking lifeless. I realized I couldn't move my arms, legs, or any part of my body except my eyes, so I began darting them around the room, trying to assess my surroundings. I was lying flat on my back on the same exam table where the testing had been done, puppy poster and all above me. At least they had positioned me correctly, I thought, since I knew that lying flat helps with blood flow when receiving epinephrine by increasing blood pressure and directing blood to the heart.

As I regained the ability to speak and hear, I noticed everyone around me was cheering. At least six people were assisting me and looking absolutely gleeful, even though I was still experiencing the scene in muffled tones like I was underwater. I was absolutely drenched in sweat, as if I had been plunged into a pool.

That's when a wave of nausea hit me, and I realized I needed to use the bathroom. I felt like I was about to be sick. They helped me up off the table and handed me a cup of oral steroid pills to swallow without water. Known in my family for being terrible at swallowing medicine, I wasn't fazed—I threw them down my throat without hesitation. That's when I realized just how *not myself* I was.

One of the first things I heard the nurse excitedly exclaim was, "You're so lucky; this was the absolute best place to go into anaphylaxis!" I stared back at her in shock, grappling with the fact that this whole ordeal had unfolded because *they* insisted I be tested for my known anaphylactic allergen. Saying I was annoyed would've been the understatement of the year.

They monitored me to make sure I didn't need a fourth epinephrine injection and warned me that a fourth epinephrine shot could induce a heart attack since epinephrine is adrenaline. Something I didn't know at the time. At that point, I was so numb to what was happening that I calmly accepted the news. They let me walk very slowly to the bathroom, but I had to leave the door open while using the toilet. Usually, I would have been embarrassed, but I wasn't even phased.

I stood up to wash my hands and gazed into my own eyes in the bathroom mirror. I pressed my fingers into the skin on my face, and it was as if I had never touched my own skin before; I couldn't tell if I was making direct contact due to the lack of sensation. My senses clearly had not fully recovered.

I could see the outer edges of my face slowly regaining their usual rosy-olive color, incrementally blending with the unrecognizable gray undertones. I looked terrible. My eyes were dark and my neck was puffy and marred by blue splotches—from the lack of oxygen—making me resemble someone who had just walked out of a zombie movie.

Learning About False-Negatives

I groggily took unsteady steps back to the same table in the allergy testing room, focusing hard on keeping my balance. The nurse informed me that the spot on my forearm where they tested me multiple times for peanuts was known for producing false negatives in skin tests. I immediately wondered why they would have tested for my life-threatening peanut allergy in that spot after I had made the severity of my condition so clear. Her casual admission left me even more bewildered, as it seemed like a glaring sign of negligence and carelessness.

In a flat, uninterested tone, she explained they'd chosen my forearm to keep the peanut test separate from the other allergens marked on my upper arms and back. But selecting a spot known for false negatives felt like a glaring oversight.

Then, without a hint of empathy, I was told that allergy shots wouldn't help my peanut allergy—or any food allergy, for that matter, as they only do them for environmental allergies. It was the first time I'd heard this. I had scheduled this entire appointment hoping for a solution to help my food allergy lessen, and very clearly explained this to them over the phone and in-person. I couldn't shake the thought: this all could've, and should've, been avoided.

Once I was comfortably back on my feet, talking and looking a little less—put bluntly—dead, they told me I was cleared to drive myself home. They guided me out, unlocking the front door, as the office had clearly been closed for a while, with me as the last lingering patient.

I got into my car and began to process what had happened. Looking at the clock, I realized that I had been there for over seven hours. When I arrived, it was lunchtime, and when I left, it was getting dark outside. The whole appointment became a blur that, in hindsight, I wished I had documented more carefully.

I immediately called my mom while sitting in my parked car in their parking lot. She was understandably horror-struck. Over the phone, she began crying, asking if they took me to a hospital. As I heard myself respond, "No," I began to realize this did seem odd.

"They didn't call an ambulance?" she asked.

"No," I told her and went on to say that I was prescribed an oral steroid to take for the next 30 days and instructed to take Benadryl regularly for at least the next five. After this reaction, I wasn't informed about the potential for additional delayed allergic reactions or any allergy testing side effects.

When I arrived back at my apartment, way later than I anticipated, I walked in to find my roommate's mom sitting on the couch. I'd only met her briefly once before, and her jaw dropped at seeing me. She rushed over with a flurry of protective, motherly concern, asking what had happened and consoling me, putting her arms on my shoulders and looking me up and down. I'd forgotten just how rough I must've looked.

Assessing myself as she held onto me, I realized I was probably stinky, wearing a damp tank top with a messy, sweat-dried top bun haphazardly pulled back, accentuating the dried blood jabbed all over my arms and back. She and I locked eyes, sharing in the same disbelief that I had driven myself home like this.

She told me that if I were one of her kids, she'd be considering a lawsuit. The thought was overwhelming; I couldn't quite process it. But seeing her so genuinely concerned gave me a sense of validation. I'd been questioning if what I'd just gone through was as traumatic as it felt—especially since the office had seemed so casual, eager to guide me out to my car and put the whole ordeal behind them.

The following day, my roommate checked in on me, and I remember the despondence in my voice, still feeling entirely out of it. I didn't know whether to feel relieved, angry, sad, or all the above. The following 30 days on oral steroids were an exhausting struggle—sleep was hard to come by, and I had to process not only the trauma of the ordeal but also the side effects of prednisone.

When I finally mustered the courage to review the

paperwork sent home with me from my allergist, I realized that I had effectively waived any claim to responsibility. Flipping through the pages and analyzing them word-for-word, I saw that I had absolved the clinic of any liability for the allergy panel and treatment I had undergone.

Regarding the cost, I paid over $800 out-of-pocket after my insurance coverage. I initially tried to dispute the balance and questioned why I wasn't taken to a hospital. Still, they refused to negotiate, stating that I had signed away all my rights in the initial office paperwork, which matched what I had read.

Although I'm not typically thinking about pursuing lawsuits, the idea crossed my mind for many years. I felt too traumatized to fully confront it, and the statute of limitations has now passed. I still have an outstanding balance of $80.00 with the office, which I don't plan to pay. The clinic informed me that I could not return unless the balance was settled, and I told them I was perfectly fine with that since I had no intention of returning to them for medical care.

This is the same clinic that conducted an oral immunotherapy trial in Louisville, but I wasn't interested in subjecting myself to further potential reactions or going back to them. As horrible as all of this was, it led me to an important realization: to never accept medical treatment that makes you uncomfortable. From this, I've learned to better advocate for myself and others and that "no" is a full sentence. This experience taught me that I have the right to refuse any medical treatment or testing that I don't want, and I encourage you to remember that you and your family do, too.

I often rely on my gut feeling when making decisions about peanuts now and allow myself space to think and not feel rushed. As my mom taught me, we know ourselves and our bodies best. Admittedly, it can be difficult to distinguish between anxiety, fear, and intuition when it comes to medical symptoms and receiving medical care.

Now, I realize that if I'm uncomfortable, I can leave and give myself time to think it over. There's no shame in putting my needs first in those situations, even if the nurses or medical staff make it seem like an unusual choice.

A Shift in Label Reading

I share this anaphylaxis story to show how others can navigate allergist experiences more safely and because it signifies a pivotal moment in my food allergy journey. This incident forced me to reevaluate how I read food labels, shaping my perspective on food allergy avoidance and safety in a whole new way.

I found over time that repeated allergic reactions increased my sensitivity to cross-contact, making me more reactive even to trace amounts of peanuts. Before 2013, I had been diligent about checking food labels for peanuts but lacked awareness of the risks posed by cross-contact, often eating products processed or potentially processed on shared equipment. I had yet to learn how drastically my approach to food would need to change.

Following my anaphylaxis episode, my allergic reactions intensified and became more frequent, highlighting the unpredictable nature of food allergies. I began reacting to foods that were likely contaminated at the facility level. Instead of just experiencing lip, neck, and chest hives with mild gastrointestinal symptoms, I faced alarming new reactions: facial numbness, eye swelling, throat constriction, and an increased reliance on antihistamines to manage these escalating reactions.

In the weeks following my anaphylactic reaction, I was driven to dive headfirst into researching food labeling laws in the US. This exploration prompted me to eliminate items that didn't specify whether peanuts were present in shared facilities. And finding this information proved to be quite challenging at first. Despite my newfound vigilance, I quickly realized the enormity of this task, but I was determined to pursue it, knowing it would be something

I'd have to do gradually. Still, it would be worth the effort to limit my reactions and finally understand their underlying cause: trace amounts of my allergen from production. It was challenging because this meant I had to inquire on each product before buying and/or eating any food item.

In 2014 and 2015, I experienced two allergic reactions from eating out, once at a restaurant and once at an extended family member's home. Both included being rushed to the hospital, receiving a steroid injection, oral medications, and hours of monitoring several vital signs and systems. That's when I decided I needed to stop eating out at restaurants or people's homes if peanuts were in their house. It was a new form of hypervigilance I'd never witnessed anyone require for a food allergy, yet it felt right. I owed it to myself to follow my gut.

I heard a lot of judgmental comments from people who felt I was being too nitpicky and overly worried. The terms "high-strung" and "high-maintenance" got tossed around. Even so, I stuck with it because I needed the change for my own well-being and was propelled to continue based on the fewer allergic reactions I experienced.

My New Protocol

The food allergy landscape has evolved significantly over the years. For some, my earlier approach of solely checking if a product intentionally contained peanuts before eating it may have seemed careless. In contrast, others might view my current method of reaching out to companies as overly extreme. Ultimately, the key is to find what works best for you and the food allergies you manage.

As Maya Angelou said, "Do the best you can until you know better. Then, when you know better, do better." I've found this wise philosophy applies to managing and living with food allergies, too. Mistakes happen, and there are countless opportunities for errors involving food allergens. Whether it's a minor oversight made in a hurry or a significant error by a company leading to a product recall, the end result can be anaphylaxis. This highlights the seriousness of food allergies: one small instance can have life-threatening consequences, regardless of how it occurs.

I often remind myself, in affirmation form, that I get to choose to surround myself with people who want to accommodate me and support me when my needs change. I want this in my friendships, and I strive to offer the same in return. Of course, people may not get it perfect every time—but it's the willingness to be supportive that truly counts. If someone alters a significant aspect of their life, I respect their decision. I know it isn't easy, and they may need support during it. In the same way, I needed support in my decision to stop eating potentially contaminated products and not accept food from others.

There was a touching line I read in the book *Uniquely Human* by Barry M. Prizant, PhD, and Tom Fields-Meyer, which explores autism as a developmental difference that affects how people communicate and experience the world. Someone on the spectrum said, "The most loving thing you can do is hear my words and believe them." Another stated, "Support us, and as things change, support us." I couldn't have said it better myself. Everyone deserves this.

Our lives are shaped by many overlapping identities that come together to make each of us unique: food allergies, celiac disease, autistic individuals, people with disabilities, LGBTQ+ folks, immigrants, children of immigrants, people of color, neurodivergent individuals, those with chronic illnesses, mental health advocates, survivors of trauma, and others. I'm filled to the brim with gratitude for today's vibrant and encouraging global food allergy community. Connecting with others who live with life-threatening food and peanut allergies—each bringing their own experiences along the allergy reactivity spectrum—has been invaluable.

Although finding transparent allergen labeling at the facility level remains a challenge in the US, I'm actively working toward labeling policy change by communicating with organizations who are also invested in this like CFAAR, FAACT, Allergy and Asthma Network, and AAFA. I also spread awareness through my *Invisibly Allergic* platforms and social circles about the transparency in allergen potential that I, and so many others, want to see from food manufacturers.

While most food manufacturers I talk to do not offer a definitive guarantee that their products are completely free of peanut contact throughout every step of the supply chain, they often state that peanuts are not used. Despite this limitation, checking with facilities has drastically helped me reduce my reactions. I recognize my privilege in managing only one anaphylactic food allergy, as handling multiple allergies requires more diligence.

Over the years, I've navigated autoimmune disease and shifting food intolerances related to it, but I am grateful to currently manage just the one peanut allergy. I understand that circumstances can change, and I never take for granted that my situation in life will remain the same. That's a lesson food allergy life has taught me.

Encouragingly, an increasing number of food brands and companies are committing to allergen-free and top 9 free facilities. Then, in 2024, I found my first allergist who listened to me and understood my food allergy experience. They validated my concerns about airborne and cross-contact reactions and addressed all my allergy questions professionally and with care. They even helped me get approved to start injectable Xolair, a drug that has been FDA-approved and used for asthma for over 20 years but is now also approved for food allergies and has the potential to reduce allergic reactions while being taken.

In closing this chapter, the word *resilience* comes to mind.

For those of us navigating the complex world of food allergies and anaphylactic shock, the end of each day is a sigh of relief in many ways. I draw strength from the stories of others who have faced similar challenges, reminding me that I am not alone.

As I continue to advocate for a safer, more understanding world for everyone affected by food allergies—facing the very real and frightening realities of anaphylaxis—I am hopeful that together we can shape a compassionate future. After experiencing this traumatic episode at the allergist's office, my family and social dynamics underwent significant changes.

Setting boundaries and asking questions about the presence of certain foods in spaces outside my homemade social navigation was particularly tricky for me, as I was asking people to do something different from before. There was a period where I often would avoid social gatherings because I didn't want to ask if they were serving food with my allergen, leaving me feeling like an outsider or a burden.

Whether it was a baby shower, a party thrown by my husband's colleague, a friend's family dinner, or a random invite to a Christmas party from an acquaintance I barely knew but wanted to get to know better, I had to ask that no peanuts be present. And communicating my needs openly and assertively wasn't easy. Sometimes the exhaustion of constantly trying to fit in tangled with my emotions, and I worried I seemed overly emotional or unclear in my ask.

My choice to stay home often surprised people if I didn't clearly explain why—I wanted to attend but couldn't because peanuts were present. Sometimes it took a few reminders for them to understand that it wasn't just a "choice" but their decision to accommodate my needs, or I couldn't come.

Food is cherished by many; people put love into it and want to share it, so my not eating it can catch them off guard, even though I want to enjoy it. I needed them to make sure anything with peanuts was removed and that their pets or kids weren't given peanut products. That didn't mean I would eat what they made, which sometimes caused tension if someone wanted me to try a special snack or cake they baked for the occasion or if it held cultural significance for their family. I'd have to explain that I try to only eat products made in peanut-free kitchens to be on the safe side.

Food is often seen as a universal language that connects people across cultures and backgrounds, but for those with food allergies, fully experiencing this connection through shared meals can be challenging, risky, and sometimes impossible. While I might not always be able to partake in traditional dishes firsthand, I find meaningful ways to engage with culture by asking for allergy-safe recipes to make at home or inviting friends over to my place to cook together using ingredients I've vetted. Beyond food, exploring culture through music, literature, storytelling, and art opens rich pathways to connection and understanding—reminding us that culture isn't just tasted, but also heard, read, and felt in many beautiful ways.

Going against the "norm" wasn't easy and sometimes felt offensive. I'd hear, "Oh, but I made this with you in mind, not using any peanuts!" As kind as that gesture was on the surface, I couldn't trust eating it since I didn't know the brands used or whether peanuts had been handled recently in the kitchen.

A few friends of mine now regularly provide safe treats and snacks for me, asking in advance about brands and my preferences for preparation, like leaving them in the original packaging. This way, I can see the label and serve myself without the risk of cross-contact, since they use my allergens in their homes when I'm not there.

Most of the time, I bring my own water bottle and safe snacks and call it a day. In the past, when I folded under pressure and chose to eat something despite the risks, I would often leave the party or event early due to a reaction, essentially putting their preference for me to eat something ahead of my preference not to have a reaction. I no longer do this.

Despite the obstacles, the years following my anaphylactic reaction have underscored the importance of self-advocacy and the value of genuine friendships rooted in mutual respect. I have learned to prioritize my health and safety, even when it means maneuvering complex misunderstandings or making tough decisions.

Closing Thoughts & Additional Context

- Prioritizing Safety in Allergy Testing: Remember to discuss the risk of anaphylactic shock from allergist office testing. Throughout this chapter, I've shared my perspective on this issue and emphasized the importance of advocating for yourself. I suggest discussing any questions or concerns with your allergist until you feel comfortable with the plan of action and to avoid feeling pressured into testing you're uncertain about. Have a plan to address this risk and be sure to discuss the potential for "false negatives" in skin tests as well. Remember, you have the right to say no and delay a procedure if you feel uncomfortable. In fact, any patient-focused doctor will tell you to do this as it's ultimately in everyone's best interest.

- Allergy Shots Won't Help Food Allergies: Allergy shots, or subcutaneous immunotherapy, are primarily designed to treat environmental allergies like pollen, dust mites, and mold, and they do not affect true food allergies. However, they can help people with Oral Allergy Syndrome (OAS), a condition where certain foods trigger allergic reactions because of cross-reactivity with pollen proteins. An ACAAI 2023 study found that roughly 50% of people with OAS who get allergy shots see improvement or even resolution of their symptoms. Importantly, there's no evidence that environmental allergy shots will cause new food allergies, making them a safe and effective option for managing OAS.

- Navigating Confusing Guidance: Sadly, some allergists still use outdated panel testing, intradermal testing, and don't clearly explain food allergies to patients. This can leave people feeling confused and avoiding foods unnecessarily, which just adds stress on top of an already challenging daily reality. Clear communication and individualized care are imperative for people with allergic conditions to understand and manage food allergies safely, and also to prevent over-generalization of food allergy experiences. Unfortunately, this is common in the food allergy space, where even people with allergic conditions sometimes assume allergies are one-size-fits-all, creating confusion for everyone—whether part of the food allergy community or not.

- Common Anaphylaxis Triggers: Anaphylactic shock can be triggered by various factors, with food being one of the most common. Our bodies have histamine receptors and other immune response pathways distributed throughout the body, therefore, anaphylaxis can produce a wide palette of symptoms. The top 9 food allergens in the US include peanuts, tree nuts, milk, eggs, fish, shellfish, soy, wheat, and sesame. In addition to food, medications and non-food products can also provoke an anaphylactic reaction due to ingredients and/or lack of ingredient transparency. Furthermore, insect stings and bites, especially from wasps and bees, are known triggers for anaphylaxis.

- Not Frequently Reported in Infants: While anaphylaxis is a potentially life-threatening allergic reaction, it is not frequently reported as a first-time reaction in infants or very young children. Research shows first-time exposures in babies result in milder symptoms, such as hives, itching (especially around the face and in the inner ears), scratching, vomiting, or general gastrointestinal upset. That said, every child is different, and it's important to recognize the early signs of a reaction, especially if they escalate quickly. Many parents understandably worry about introducing allergenic foods, but it's worth knowing that anaphylactic reactions in infancy are rare. Awareness doesn't have to equal fear, it can just mean being prepared and having a plan in place with your pediatrician or allergist.

- Seeking Support and Acknowledging Sensitivity: This chapter explored the profound realities of living with life-threatening allergies, highlighting the risks of anaphylaxis and the emotional toll these experiences can take. I recognize that these topics can be triggering and sensitive subjects for some readers, so it's essential to approach them with care and compassion. Navigating these intense situations requires not only personal self-compassion but also the empathy of those around you. Remember, it's perfectly okay to prioritize your well-being. Chapter 11 will delve deeper into the relationship between food allergies and mental health, further exploring how to navigate these complex emotional landscapes.

5

LIFE AFTER ANAPHYLAXIS: FINDING HUMOR AND HEALING

Setting Boundaries and Finding Lightness

The five personal stories in this chapter follow my ongoing journey to set clear food allergy boundaries—with friends, family, and, most importantly, myself. Developing the confidence to communicate my needs instead of giving in to my instinct to people-please hasn't come easily. Still, it's been an essential part of my healing. Self-advocacy may always be a challenge for me, and that's okay because growth doesn't look the same for everyone.

Over the last decade, attending therapy has helped me see how prioritizing others has been my way of avoiding my own emotional needs. This insight has brought both clarity and new challenges for me. Each story in this chapter captures moments of learning, mixing humor and joy with the occasional chaos of food allergy life. It's not all doom and gloom—food allergies have led me to unexpected romances, plenty of laughs, and more than a few memorable party stories. As I share here, these experiences remind me that despite difficulties, there's room for connection.

A few of my strongest friendships initially became strained by food allergy discussions that didn't go as planned when I was in my 20s. Due to my sudden change in needs after learning about the lack of labeling laws, I was referred to as "high-strung," "needy," "paranoid," and generally just misunderstood. Over time, though, as my friends gained a deeper understanding of my evolving needs, those bonds were mended. Their acceptance came with a genuine desire to accommodate, and in turn, it opened new opportunities for me to better support them in their own lives.

This chapter explores how hard experiences often ended in

shared happiness and even unexpected closeness and laughter. Embracing humor has helped me immensely, not taking life too seriously, even as food allergies add their own unique and intense twist to life's journey.

Here you'll find lighthearted stories that aim to bring a smile to your face and hopefully make you laugh alongside me as I share the quirks and insights that have come with managing my peanut allergy. As friends and family showed interest in understanding my evolving allergy and its impact on my daily life, I became more comfortable sharing the often-overlooked details of my food allergy thought process and routines.

These glimpses provided them with a valuable allergy context while assisting me in knowing what is most helpful to share with others. This openness revealed a new side of my life with food allergies, showing that not everything has to be so serious. While anaphylaxis is a real concern, it's also okay to simultaneously find joy in moments when we can forget about our allergies.

As someone who greatly values vulnerability in all aspects, it's only fair to share my own moments of vulnerable awkwardness. So, buckle up! What I'm about to recount is my experience trudging the perilous world of "What can I eat?" right after experiencing my anaphylactic reaction. If you have a food allergy, you likely relate to that lost feeling when trying to find safe foods to eat after a new or changed allergy diagnosis.

This newfound uncertainty came after my anaphylactic reaction at the allergist, forcing me to completely rethink the food choices I'd been making over two decades as I paved a new way to eat safely.

The Time I Juiced 6 Beets

In the aftermath of my terrifying allergic reaction, I felt like I was in a state of disbelief and at the same time, relieved, simply grateful to be alive. My body was still reeling from the effects of anaphylactic shock, battling hives, mild swelling, and the quirky side effects of taking a hefty dose of steroids like insomnia. The reality was that I was afraid to eat.

While I've never had an eating disorder, I believe that in the weeks after my reaction, I came close to understanding how it might feel, especially when someone is trying to manage food allergies or similar. My fear of eating anything potentially contaminated with peanuts was overwhelming; I didn't want to risk triggering another reaction in my already stressed-out system. To play it safe, I opted for a diet of natural, unprocessed foods like fruits, vegetables, whole grains, and healthy fats. This approach seemed the best way to avoid any hidden peanut contamination and help my body recover.

Among my new food choices, beets became a particular focus. An Ayurvedic cookbook I'd recently read touted beets as nutrient-rich, anti-inflammatory, and great for digestion. I took this advice to heart and bought a whole, literal bunch of large red beets.

Beets—whether roasted or raw—were never something I craved. But hey, I figured, I'm eating healthy, so I might as well give them another shot. Plus, their vibrant color was appealing. As I cut into them, I could literally see how they were bursting with nutrients! I dusted off my juicer, which I rarely use because it's a pain to clean and I proceeded to make a seemingly nourishing juice for myself. I was ready to feel revitalized from the power of beets!

With anticipation, I scrolled through my phone for a beet juice recipe. Most included celery and apples—ingredients I don't particularly enjoy. Carrots and herbs would have been ideal, but I didn't have any. So, I kept it simple: I juiced the beets with half of an organic lemon and called it a day.

Surprisingly, I didn't completely hate it! With a straw sticking directly into the pitcher, I plopped down in front of the TV, ready to sip my way to good health. But as the juice turned from a refreshing sip into a bit of a chore, I thought, forget it, I'm chugging this thing and following it up with some water. I gulped down the juice, chased it with a big swig of water, and almost immediately, my stomach churned. I felt a hot sensation creeping up from my chest to my neck and next to my face. Uh-oh, was this an allergic reaction? I started to panic and dashed to my room to grab my epinephrine.

Next, I bolted to the bathroom. Ready to confront my cramping stomach, but nothing happened. Instead, I stared at my beet-red cheeks in the mirror, not from the juice staining my skin but from the heat brewing underneath. It was as if my body was asking me sternly, "What did you just do to me?"

I knew quickly that my discomfort wasn't an allergic reaction but rather the result of chugging the juice of 6 enormous beets in record time. Whoops. While sitting on the toilet, I took out my phone and Googled the recommended amount of beet juice. It turns out that the usual starting point is to juice one medium-sized beet, which is about two inches in diameter. Well, I'd juiced more than eight times, given my beets were closer to three inches each. *Cool, cool, cool.* My stomach had much to say about it, gurgling loud enough to make me look down and hold it in surprise.

I read on, and the internet helpfully informed me that beet juice is quite potent and typically diluted with other juices or water. *Excellent*, I thought. I definitely *hadn't* done that. Meanwhile, I remained stationed in the bathroom, though nothing much was happening—just my stomach's continuing murmuring, probably heard by my roommates several rooms away.

After about 45 minutes, my skin had cooled down, so I finally ventured out of the bathroom and decided to Google "constipation from beet juice." Lo and behold, I discovered that consuming too much beet juice can indeed overwhelm your digestive system and lead to constipation. How delightful.

There you have it—I've definitely overshared, and I hope for your sake that you never consume close to an equivalent amount of raw beet juice in one sitting. To this day, the mere thought of juicing a beet sends a shiver down my spine; I can feel goosebumps prickling along my arms as I cringe just from thinking about it.

In all seriousness, though, when navigating new allergies or dietary restrictions, focusing on simple, wholesome elements—and really savoring them—can be surprisingly rewarding. Things like fresh fruit, plain rice with simple seasoning, or a nourishing broth can taste incredibly satisfying, especially compared to heavily processed foods.

After going through my elimination diet, fruits tasted so sweet, almost like a dessert—such a shift in perspective! Of course, if your allergies include fruits or rice, you can focus on other safe options. The key is to embrace what you can have, even if it feels "too boring" at first. That boredom is normal while you figure out your new food landscape, but it will pass. Your taste buds will adjust, and before long, you'll rediscover joy in eating again.

It's often much harder for adults to navigate a food allergy diagnosis compared to kids, because adults have to change lifelong habits, while kids tend to adapt more naturally. For example, I've never had peanut butter, so I don't miss it or have a reference point of it, but someone who grew up loving it might feel more grief. The good news is, it gets better as you learn your boundaries and find enjoyable ways to eat around them.

Powdery Poison

By the mid-2010s, powdered peanut butter had suddenly become a household and smoothie bar staple. It seemed like overnight it was popping up in every grocery store and health food shop, touted as a lower-fat, lower-calorie alternative to regular peanut butter. The appeal was clear for many: an easy protein boost for smoothies, breakfast bowls, a quick umami addition to savory foods, and more. I guess I get it.

But for those of us with peanut allergies—especially airborne ones—powdered PB felt like a new nightmare unlocked. At least, that's how it hit me. I've had more than my fair share of run-ins with this powdery poison, but the most memorable incident that comes to mind involved an entire shelf collapsing in my local grocery store, with me "lucky" enough to be right there. I came out of it fine, but I won't lie; it felt like the universe had created a dramatic spectacle just for me. Because as I find myself saying a bit too often for comfort, what are the odds?

Picture this: I had gone to a store that I frequented occasionally but wasn't entirely familiar with in terms of layout because it wasn't in my neighborhood. I aimed to quickly grab a few items and move on to my other nearby errands. Given that I'm always on high alert in grocery stores, where food allergens tend to lurk, I cautiously navigated the produce section as usual.

As I turned my shopping cart into an aisle stocked with soda cans and snacks, I noticed something odd on the floor—chalky, ghostly footprints and cart tracks zigzagged around in an off-white powder. My curiosity was piqued, but unsure of what it was, I did my best to avoid it, stepping cautiously to stay on clean patches of the floor—reminding me of the childhood game "The Floor Is Lava."

I continued, slowly rounding the corner into the next aisle, only to find it strewn with open canisters of powder. *Aha, there's the culprit*, I thought, assuming it was some type of dish detergent powder. But then, my heart sank as I spotted the "protein powder" aisle marker. Uh oh. Then I saw it—about fifty opened and spilled powdered peanut butter containers, creating a small mountain of powdered PB on the floor.

I had no idea how it had happened, but it was clear the employees were aware, as there was a single orange cone marking the disaster zone. I abandoned my grocery cart faster than I could scream *peanut dust!* and made a beeline for the front exit within my view, my senses on high alert and my heart racing. I was running and holding my breath, zigzagging around people and their carts as if running for escape in a disaster movie.

The automatic doors struggled to keep pace with my frantic exit, but I slipped through, desperately searching for any surface to wipe my contaminated shoes on while gulping in fresh air. In the distance, I spotted a small patch of grass and sprinted toward it, rubbing the soles of my shoes against the concrete and sandy gravel as I passed. I'm sure it looked confusing and alarming to onlookers.

I did my best to clean my shoes on the grass without wet wipes handy, shifting to fresh spots for thoroughness. As I caught my breath from running, it dawned on me how dangerous the situation could have been—and still was—for others with peanut allergies inside. I took my time, monitoring my breathing and doing a body scan to check for any signs of an allergic reaction. Finding none, I took an Alavert as a precaution, relieved to have avoided what could have been a particularly severe situation. I was still in shock from it all. I attempted to call the store, but after waiting on hold with their automated system for a while, I decided to continue my errands.

Whenever I share this story, I can't help but shake my head at its sheer absurdity, but also at the reality it reveals. For me, it wasn't just bizarre; it was a reminder of how quickly something as ordinary as a trip to the grocery store can turn into a fight for safety.

My $25 Groupon Tattoo

No one warned me not to make major life decisions while on a high dose of steroids. So, I'm sharing this story with you. Consider it a public service announcement. You're welcome!

In the past, I've been prescribed 30-day rounds of steroids a couple of times due to my food allergy and autoimmune disease, in order to calm my immune response and reduce inflammation. And to be clear, I haven't ended up with a new tattoo or made any other drastic decisions since the first time.

However, drug interactions can be unpredictable, and you never know how they might affect you, so it's best to proceed tentatively. Here's the $25 Groupon tattoo story you never knew you wanted to hear—and that you most certainly didn't ask for.

After my anaphylactic reaction at the allergist's office, I was frustratingly struck with insomnia and irregular sleep cycles. Despite practicing relaxation techniques before bed and taking the steroid early each morning with breakfast, it didn't go away. The first week wasn't too bad, but by weeks two and three, the sleep deprivation began to take its toll. That's when I found myself aimlessly browsing and shopping online in the middle of the night, hopping from site to site to pass the time.

One early morning—or late night, depending on your perspective—while struggling to sleep with my glazed-over eyes wide open, I got a pop-up advertising Groupon in my area. I followed it, and it took me to a nearby tattoo parlor with prices starting at just $25. Excitedly, I bought a voucher for a 2" by 4" placement I'd envisioned for months—what a steal! In hindsight, seeking a cheap deal for something permanent might not be the best idea, but I was too thrilled to care. With the purchase, I had to pick my scheduled time. Having just narrowly escaped death and experienced a life-altering event, I felt invigorated and ready to embrace life to the fullest. *Should I finally get that tattoo I've been dreaming of?*

Absolutely. *Carpe diem.* For a moment I wondered, *should I get the phrase "carpe diem" tattooed on me?* But my friends knew I had a particular phrase in mind inspired by one of my favorite artists.

A week later, my closest friends accompanied me to my appointment. Enthusiasm buzzed in the air as we walked together, practically hip to hip, carried along by our own excitement. The neighborhood's pulse matched our own, with businesses spilling music from open doors and strangers brushing past, and we fit right into its rhythm on the way to the parlor.

But as soon as we walked in, the mood shifted. The place looked uninviting and grim, and the tattoo artist began rambling, muttering something strange and slightly offensive. I couldn't tell whether it made sense, whether he was joking, or maybe both.

A nagging feeling crept in that I might regret this decision. But I was already there, and I'd already paid. Once again, I was faced with the lesson of learning to say no and leave if something feels wrong...*sigh*. I should have taken the $25 price tag as a warning, but I didn't. Can you see where this is going?

Years later, I learned from a more skilled tattoo artist that my original artist's heavy-handed approach left deep, lasting marks. While I didn't dislike the tattoo itself and liked its placement, the text was drawing unwanted attention from strangers who would randomly touch it or ask to see it closer. Ultimately, that unwanted, awkward magnetic attention pushed me to have it removed.

After more than 30 expensive laser treatments, it's now gone, but the scar tissue and hypopigmentation left behind will always remind me of that $25 anaphylaxis-driven, steroid-fogged decision. I've now gained a *profound* appreciation for a skilled tattoo artist with a light hand!

Now, whenever I'm told I need to take steroids, my mind goes straight back to my infamous Groupon experience. Instead of 'roid rage, I got 'roid remorse. This experience serves as a little cautionary tale to remind me to be extra careful about my mental and physical health while on corticosteroids—or, really, any strong prescription. These meds can do a number on anxiety or agitation; they can mess with sleep and focus, too, sometimes leading to...well, choices like a $25 permanent decision. Just a candid story of a questionable decision after nearly dying and a week of no sleep. What a ride!

The "Under the Table" Comment

Typically, the phrase "under the table" hints at something done secretly. For me, though, it now holds a dual meaning. And trust me, if you've been through enough bad medical experiences to feel a little jaded, this is a story you'll want to hear.

In 2017, I visited an allergist who came highly recommended by an acquaintance in Louisville. She trusted this allergist to manage her child's life-threatening food allergies, so I felt conservatively optimistic. This was my first time in an allergist's office since the last time when I had my 2013 reaction, and I was ready to share my experience living with a lifelong peanut allergy, including reactions to airborne and cross-contact exposures, and get some advice on how to best manage it. Except, before I could start explaining my allergy history, the allergist cut me off.

"Let me stop you right there—" he interrupted, puffing out his chest and sitting taller to emphasize his authority. Without waiting for a response, he launched into a story about another allergist he knew who would smear peanut butter under the tables of patients claiming airborne allergies, to "test" and debunk them to their faces. He said he had even considered doing the same "test" himself. My eyes went wide, my brain short-circuited, and I think I opened my mouth as if to say something but couldn't because I was *horrified*. He didn't react, either not noticing or not caring.

When I tried to explain that the allergen would likely need to be ingested and then exhaled nearby, or become airborne as peanut dust, like from someone shaking an open bag of roasted peanuts into their hands and then dusting off their hands into the air, he ignored me and shifted topics without missing a beat. He reached over and touched both my earlobes, startling me slightly, then smiled widely and loudly asked about my piercings and whether I had any metal sensitivities.

Confused and disheartened, I thought, *okay…this allergist visit is not going as I'd hoped.* Amidst his nonstop chatter, I managed to squeeze in quickly, "Yes, I do. Though my ears are pierced, I can't wear earrings often because they get hot and inflamed." Upon hearing this, he straightened proudly, declaring, "I thought so—

that's common with peanut allergies!" Clapping his hands together, he seemed to have a look of *Voilà, my work here is done!* While I reluctantly admitted that this was an interesting connection, I couldn't help but feel frustrated; I hadn't even started sharing my detailed medical history with him, and he showed no interest in what I had to say or what was written on the piece of paper I brought with me.

He continued with a long-winded monologue, dismissing all airborne food allergies as nonexistent. When I raised concerns about inadequate US food labeling laws, he brushed them aside, steering the conversation as he pleased. Although I used his services that day to order a comprehensive blood panel to compare with my 2013 results, which I took to LabCorp, I never returned to his office.

I knew that if I ever needed an allergist again, I'd have to continue my search—preferably for someone willing to hear my story, respect my experiences, and show genuine interest in helping their patients. Medical gaslighting, which ties directly into my experience above, can look many ways. It can be the dismissal of symptoms, a lack of curiosity, or medical professionals not being open-minded simply because they have not personally seen a certain presentation before.

I believe in evidence-based medical care, and in clinicians who are honest about what we know, what we do not know yet, and where research is still developing. Just because something is unfamiliar to a provider does not mean it isn't real or worthy of care. There is no single blueprint for how conditions show up in different bodies. Part of my goal with this book is to equip others with information so they can better advocate for themselves, feel more in control when seeking care, and encourage open-mindedness in medicine to help reduce medical gaslighting—especially for those navigating allergies and allergic conditions, menopause and perimenopause, chronic conditions, and more.

Mixed Nuts and Marriage Material

I never expected that having an allergic reaction on a date just a month in would reveal so much about the person I was newly seeing.

I was anticipating it would be an easy, carefree night. I'd ordered takeout from a family-owned restaurant just down the street—a place I'd frequented dozens of times and considered one of my "regular" spots. Since I'd already spoken with them multiple times about my peanut allergy, explicitly asking about peanuts and peanut oil, I felt confident they didn't use any in their kitchen.

That night, I strolled into The Falafel House, a little more dressed up than usual and feeling excited. I ordered my favorite hummus platter with extra pita, and on a whim, I decided to grab a dessert I hadn't tried before. I knew Paul, the guy I was going on dates with, loved baklava, and I noticed they had it on the menu. I asked if any peanuts were in it, and they confidently reassured me it was a mix of walnuts and pistachios—*no peanuts*. Although I don't recall the exact conversation, I left with the impression that peanuts still weren't used in anything at the restaurant. Since I'd often eaten there safely, I felt comfortable trusting their answer.

I headed back to my apartment, where Paul was waiting. As soon as we sat down to eat, I revealed my baklava surprise, even suggesting we start with dessert. Growing up, my mom encouraged starting with dessert, calling it the best part—and I wholeheartedly agree. Why save the best for last, or get too full and miss out completely?

I pulled the plastic clamshell container from the bag, opened it, and handed Paul a plastic fork. Leaning in to smell the baklava, I caught a faint peanut-like scent but reassured myself internally by recalling the staff's promise: *no peanuts*. Trusting their word, I took a tiny lick—instantly, I knew. There *were* peanuts.

Panic set in as I dashed to the bathroom, shouting behind me as I ran, "There are peanuts in this!" As I flushed my mouth with water and took an antihistamine, I could feel that the reaction was escalating. Returning to the room, I told him urgently, "We need to get to immediate care or the hospital right now." He nodded, stepping into action. Though he knew about my allergy, he didn't yet know all the details I usually save for later. I wasn't sure if he'd even thought about my EpiPens. Almost as if reading my mind, he asked where they were. I grabbed my bag with them inside, and we bolted down the stairs from my second-floor apartment.

I can't recall if we took his car or mine, but he drove as I sat with my EpiPens in my lap. "If the reaction worsens and you need the injection, just tell me—I'll do it," he reassured me. As he drove, I struggled through the panic, trying to decide between the ER and urgent care. The ER was slightly closer, but I worried about the cost.

Ultimately, I chose urgent care—a place I trusted with a specific doctor I liked, about nine minutes away. I'd already taken the antihistamines at the first signs of lip swelling and tingling, and I kept taking one every few minutes as we drove. I monitored my symptoms carefully in case we needed to use my epinephrine autoinjector.

He sped through the streets with intense focus, navigating swiftly and purposefully to get me to urgent care quickly and safely. I knew he was a self-proclaimed "car guy," but now I could see his knack for handling high-speed maneuvers in action and that he took pride in his driving skills. It worked in my favor, and I was impressed.

When we arrived, he let me out at the entrance doors and went to park the car. I rushed to the front desk, urgently explaining that I was having an allergic reaction to peanuts and possibly experiencing anaphylaxis. They immediately took me to the back and started treatment. The medical team was alarmed by the number of antihistamines I had taken—almost more alarmed than the reaction itself! This caught me off guard.

As I'd hoped, my usual doctor was on duty, and I had complete trust in her as she had helped me in multiple instances over the years. I told her I had taken 8 Benadryl and was still feeling the reaction intensify, though I wasn't struggling to breathe—just dealing with mild swelling and hives. So, I didn't know if I should use my epinephrine.

I've covered this in other parts of the book, but it bears repeating: taking such high doses of Benadryl or any antihistamine is not advisable. As I said before, this was my method of self-medicating and managing reactions for a long time, before I learned antihistamines could mask symptoms of anaphylaxis and should not be taken in excessive amounts. For anaphylaxis, the best approach is to use epinephrine promptly if you think you may need it. But back to the story—

They got me into an open exam room, which was luckily available, and administered a steroid shot in my thigh while closely monitoring my vital signs and symptoms. This is another thing that's changed in the medical field from this reaction to now. I used to be given steroid shots at urgent care and the ER for peanut reactions, but now it's advised to provide epinephrine instead. It's still something that is trickling down in terms of information in the medical field with early adopters and laggards and so on, but that's something I've heard from many board-certified allergists to advocate for yourself for if you're in a situation where the medical staff is wanting to give a steroid shot versus epinephrine for a food allergy response. Epinephrine should be the go-to.

Paul waited anxiously, pacing between the waiting room and hallway area while I received the injection. During this time, I began experiencing stomach gurgles and knew I was about to be hit with gastrointestinal issues that commonly come with a reaction.

The medical team wasn't sure if these symptoms were due

to the peanut exposure or the large number of antihistamines I had taken. Regardless, I used their bathroom on and off as I started feeling better, and the swelling subsided. To ensure my safety in case of any worsening reaction, they had me leave the bathroom door slightly ajar without locking it. I was grateful that my new date wasn't right by my side during this, as I was feeling embarrassed.

Once I was back in the exam room, the nurse came by to check on me, and I felt much better. She smiled and said, "Girl, you need to take this man to the courthouse after this; he really cares about you." Surprised, I looked at her, and she explained how, unbeknownst to me, Paul had been checking in, trying to be respectful and not hover.

She got the context since I'd mentioned we were on a date. At first, I was taken aback, thinking, *Huh? The courthouse?* But, as the sweetness of her comment sank in, I couldn't help but smile. That definitely went in the "pros" column; he really did seem like a genuinely caring person.

While I didn't immediately carry out the nurse's courthouse suggestion, I definitely appreciated her kind words. I could tell that Paul's calm, reassuring presence had impressed her—and I had to agree. He handled the situation incredibly well, especially considering it was his first time witnessing an allergic reaction and knowing he might need to use my epinephrine. Even though I was the one experiencing the reaction, he could tell I was scared—something I'm still working on in therapy due to having an aversion to needles. It put me at ease to know that he was ready and willing to administer the medication if I couldn't do it myself, offering the kind of support I needed most.

In hindsight, her comment was prophetic. We're married now and have been for almost a decade! Looking back, I loved his caring response during that moment and the way afterward he consistently handled my food allergy day-to-day—it matched so many of my core values.

A little over a year later, I ended up back at that same urgent care for an unrelated issue, and I got to share with her that we were engaged. She remembered me and even recalled a few details from that day. She mentioned that she had a family member named Zoë, which is why my name had stuck with her—a small but meaningful connection that added to the story.

So, there is my little romantic urgent care story! Looking back, it's cute since it had a happy ending, and I sometimes forget it happened now that so much time has passed. But in that moment, it really showed me how much of a stand-up person my date was. Here's some advice: if you're with someone who doesn't handle your allergy respectfully and with importance, move on. There are kind people out there who will take your needs seriously—and we all deserve that!

Closing Thoughts & Additional Context

- Antihistamines Can Mask Anaphylaxis Symptoms: It took me years to fully grasp how crucial it is to use epinephrine during a severe allergic reaction, partly because I was afraid of the needle and partly because it's expensive to replace. I've since learned that over-the-counter drugs like antihistamines can be dangerously misleading in a crisis. First-generation antihistamines, such as diphenhydramine (Benadryl), can cause sedation and impair cognitive function, potentially masking symptoms of anaphylaxis and delaying the administration of epinephrine.

- Antihistamines vs. Epinephrine: Second-generation antihistamines, like cetirizine (Zyrtec), loratadine (Claritin), and fexofenadine (Allegra) are less sedating, but they are still not suggested for treating anaphylaxis. Many people say nothing works as well as Benadryl, which makes sense if it helps with symptoms—but this is just good information to have in your back pocket, regardless of whether you prefer to use first- or second-generation antihistamines. They may mask the symptoms of anaphylactic shock and delay your dosing of the life-saving drug epinephrine. So, here's the key takeaway: if you actively experience symptoms affecting multiple body systems—skin reactions, respiratory distress, or gastrointestinal symptoms—don't hesitate to use epinephrine immediately. It's the most effective treatment, and there's no medical downside to using it.

- Emotional Challenges: Communicating the severity of food allergies whether in medical settings, work, or personal relationships—can be an emotional experience. I've felt misunderstood and defensive when navigating these conversations if I get the sense that a person feels I'm overreacting. These challenging interactions taught me to assert my needs more effectively. But I'm still not perfect at it; depending on my mood and mental health, my emotions can vary widely across different situations. Recently, I discovered Cognitive Behavioral Therapy (CBT) for managing food allergy anxiety and trauma, and I'm excited to explore it further. Food allergy anxiety is part of the allergy experience, and having tools like CBT could make a significant difference in processing and responding in these heightened moments.

- Use Caution with Steroids: In this chapter, I shared a humorous yet cautionary tale about my impulsive choice while on corticosteroids. Although it's funny in hindsight, it highlights the real side effects of certain medications and the need for careful decisions during treatment—something that doctors or pharmacists don't always discuss enough. Side effects like sleeplessness and mood changes can be serious, especially with long-term steroid use, and deserve attention. Speaking with a medical professional about potential side effects and asking questions upfront can help prepare for any symptoms and offer valuable guidance. With some extra knowledge, avoiding these effects is more manageable than reacting to them.

- Why Advocacy Matters in Medicine: My experience with the dismissive allergist further underscores the need for self-advocacy in healthcare, especially when dealing with complex and often misunderstood topics and conditions. Finding an allergist who genuinely understands and supports your needs can be a time-consuming and expensive journey requiring patience, persistence, and energy. However, it's worth it for effective allergy management and peace of mind. To anyone searching for a medical professional who truly listens and connects with you, know you're not alone. Sending love and support to everyone in that process—it's challenging, but finding the proper care for you can make all the difference!

- Therapeutic Insights: Talk therapy has been instrumental in helping me balance avoiding allergens while fully living my life. It has also allowed me to find lightheartedness in intense situations, such as allergic reactions, enabling me to move on without being overwhelmed by repeated anxiety or constantly reliving the experience in a fight-or-flight state. I view therapy as something lifelong that I'll do on and off indefinitely, not just for my food allergy but for myself in general. As I've learned from Dr. Nadine Burke Harris' talks on our bodily stress system, which I discuss more in Chapter 11, our stress response—fight, flight, and freeze—evolved to keep us alive. She describes it as "like a finely tuned Swiss watch where every part affects the whole. When in balance, it can save our lives; when disrupted by repeated or intense adversity, it can shorten them." Understanding this has helped me see why talk therapy has been so important in balancing allergen avoidance with fully living my life. In addition to the classic fight-or-flight response, research shows that many people also respond to stress with a "tend-and-befriend" approach, leaning on connection, care, and support from others, which can be a powerful complement to practical coping strategies.

- Neffy: Painful, But Effective: I used the Neffy nasal spray epinephrine during a recent anaphylaxis episode at a restaurant, which I suspect was a cross-contact reaction—likely from cheese contaminated by peanuts during preparation or at the facility level. I double-checked the restaurant's allergen binder with the manager and confirmed that no peanuts were used in their kitchen. Despite the burning and nasal discomfort, it worked and administered easily. I would use it again in a similar situation, though I'm not sure I'd recommend it for children unless you can warn them about the potential for long-lasting pain. One month after using it, I was still experiencing nasal sensitivity and inflammation in the nostril where it was administered, and I found myself unusually aware of that area. After two months, I ended up needing a prescription antibiotic for my nose, which resolved the lingering sensations. Since Neffy is so new, I'm not sure if my experience is typical. I did report it to the company, and my allergist documented it as part of their ongoing data collection, since none of their other patients had tried it yet. What I appreciate most about a needle-free option is that I didn't hesitate to use it the way I have with my auto-injector, due to fear of needles or having to push it through my clothes, and extreme temperatures don't impact it as much as traditional needle medications. I value having this option, but wish there was more awareness from the manufacturer about what to expect in terms of face pain and discomfort. I hope needle-free alternatives become more accessible and affordable for everyone.

6

DECODING FOOD LABELS

Cracking the Code: How I Read Food Labels

Unfortunately navigating food labels can sometimes feel like decoding a foreign language. This section explains my simple method for reading US food labels for top allergens. Surprisingly, this topic gets less attention in the food allergy space than you might expect but understanding how to read labels is primarily how I avoid having allergic reactions.

Despite my numerous inquiries to medical professionals, I have never received this kind of guidance from an allergist or doctor. Alarmingly, I often find myself educating doctors and allergists about the glaring inadequacies in our food labeling laws concerning allergen requirements. Every allergist I've seen—except my most recent—was unaware that "may contain" statements are voluntary, undefined, and not mandated. This highlights the enormous gaps in allergy education within the medical field. While progress is being made, it's clear we still have a long way to go. Especially when it comes to ingredients that fall outside of the top 9 most common allergens.

While the method I've developed has dramatically reduced my own allergic reactions, it's not a one-size-fits-all solution. Everyone's food allergies, reactions, and preferences are unique, so I hope this information can inspire you to craft your own effective food label reading strategy. In this chapter, I've broken the process into quick, straightforward steps for you to follow.

To start, I need to lay the groundwork with a brief overview. If a product intentionally contains any of the top 9 allergens, the FDA must clearly list them on the ingredient label in a way that stands out. The unfortunate thing is that even with these protections, recalls can still happen. Also, this doesn't account for trace amounts of allergens from shared facilities or shared lines. It's important to note that these requirements are limited to food products. They do not include labeling the top 9 allergens in non-food items such as skin and body products, cosmetics, household products, supplements, alcoholic beverages, or medications.

In fact, a proposed act in Congress called the, "Allergen Disclosure In Non-food Articles Act" or the "ADINA Act", aims to expand FDA labeling requirements to mandate the clear, transparent labeling of major food allergens and gluten in over the counter and prescription medications in the United States. Many might assume this type of labeling is already required, but it's not.

I've heard horror stories of individuals suffering anaphylactic reactions to prescription medications like steroids and antibiotics containing top allergens such as lactose, which is derived from milk. This is alarming, as steroids are often prescribed to patients after experiencing anaphylaxis, so if someone has a dairy allergy and experiences anaphylaxis and then is prescribed a steroid that unknowingly contains dairy derivatives... You can see how this could be especially dangerous.

It's also important for individuals undergoing fertility treatments or other hormonal therapies to be aware that some medications, such as lipid emulsions or progesterone capsules, may contain oils or ingredients derived from peanut, sesame, soy, egg, or other common allergens. Many of these hormones are delivered in oil-based solutions, which is why allergenic oils are sometimes used as carriers. These components can cause unexpected allergic reactions, so it's crucial to discuss any known sensitivities with your healthcare provider and carefully check ingredient lists before starting treatment.

As it stands, people with food allergies can easily spend multiple hours with pharmacists trying to determine if their allergens are present in their prescriptions or not, which is time-consuming and inefficient for all parties involved. The ADINA Act would be an incredible feat if passed, though it would not cover vitamins or supplements because those aren't regulated by the FDA under the specific act they're seeking to amend, so that's an important detail to note. For tracking legislation related to food allergies and other issues, Congress.gov is a valuable resource for checking the status of federal bills, identifying supporting representatives, and receiving legislative updates. Hopefully, this resource will continue to be available, even with the current administration.

For state-level legislation, you'll need to look at each state legislature's website, but there are tools that make this process much easier. LegiScan offers a user-friendly way to track bills across all 50 states, providing alerts and summaries that save time and effort. You'll need to create a free account to access the tracking features, but the setup is quick and well worth it. Using LegiScan can help streamline the often overwhelming task of staying informed about legislation that directly affects daily life with food allergies.

Circling back to food labeling requirements, if you have one take away from this chapter let it be this: When you see any type of "may contain" or "in a shared facility with" allergy statement on a product or even a prominent "nut-free" logo, understand that these are entirely unregulated. These labels are known as Precautionary Allergen Labeling (PAL) claims. PAL refers to allergens that may unintentionally enter a product through shared equipment or shared facilities, not ingredients that are deliberately added to the formula. This distinction matters because PAL warnings are about possible cross-contact risk rather than intentional formulation.

There are no mandates or monitoring to ensure PAL accuracy or define their meanings. Because of this, any such claims on products, including references to allergens at the facility level, should always be cautiously approached. Many people with and without allergies are often surprised to learn this.

Sharing and revealing the gaps in our labeling protections can be overwhelming as an allergic person and food allergy advocate. The sad reality is that I wish our laws were more robust and comprehensive. Even with a life-threatening peanut allergy, I've had to create my own framework for eating. This is because trying to find the information I need to make simple food choices is time-consuming, often leading to dead ends and uncertain answers from food brands I've inquired about to see if I can safely eat their products.

There are times I knowingly eat products without being certain about the allergens present in the facility. I try to avoid this as much as possible, but living with a food allergy means making educated guesses and taking calculated risks daily based on available information. It's like dining at restaurants that don't actively use my allergen, but likely source ingredients from facilities that do, where there could be trace peanut amounts.

Living with a life-threatening allergy means every decision is a calculated risk. Even when a product is labeled 100% peanut-free, a part of me remains skeptical—what if an employee brought an allergen into the space and contaminated ingredients without anyone knowing? This constant vigilance means I'm always prepared for a reaction and never fully confident I won't have one. Yet, when I don't react, there's a quiet celebration.

The process I use to manage my food allergy took me a long time to fully commit to. If a doctor had advised me to follow these steps, I likely would have taken it more seriously right away. But because I assigned this undertaking to myself, it took me a few years to stick with it. Between 2013 and 2016, fewer food allergy Facebook groups, Instagram accounts, or apps like Spokin were available than today. Without a reliable allergist to consult, I had to develop this set of rules based on what I understood about my body.

As I mentioned, our labeling law issues extend beyond the foods we eat to non-food items, which I'll explore further in the following chapter. But as promised, let's dive into how to easily decode food ingredient labels.

My Process for Reading US Food Labels

Understanding food labels can be overwhelming, especially with food allergies or conditions like celiac disease. Over the years, I've developed a 3-step process to help ensure products are safe for me. If I can't find the allergen information I need, I usually skip it—but for rare finds, I'll purchase the product and do this later. Here's my approach:

Step 1: Examine the Ingredient Label Thoroughly

Whether in a store or browsing a food product online, I closely examine the product name and locate the ingredient label—often reading it multiple times over—to ensure it doesn't contain my allergen.

In the US, the Food Allergen Labeling and Consumer Protection Act (FALCPA) mandates that the top 9 food allergens must be clearly listed if they are ingredients in a food product. Using scientific or Latin terms like "arachis oil" instead of "peanut" is not permitted because it would make allergen identification confusing and unsafe for consumers. Meaning, the word "peanut" must be used to identify its presence. The only exception is if an allergen is a "refined" oil, then the FDA exempts this from needing to be called out explicitly.

Step 2: Check for Facility-Level Allergen Statements

Next, I look for any Precautionary Allergen Labeling (PAL) statements on the packaging, such as "This product is made in a facility with soy, wheat, and eggs" or "This product was made in a peanut and tree nut-free facility." If the product is made in a facility without my allergens, I personally choose to trust this information and will consider purchasing it. It's worth noting these statements are not mandatory, regulated, or checked for accuracy.

These statements can sometimes be hidden in logos or on the front of the packaging, so it requires some detective work. There is no standardized format for these claims.

Speaking from my own experience, it is quite frustrating that PAL statements are not regulated in the US. This means companies are not legally required to include them, and their use can vary widely between brands and products. As a result, the presence or absence of PAL doesn't guarantee an item's safety, which can be confusing and often leads to uncertainty for consumers who rely on these statements. It's a tricky situation—I greatly appreciate PAL information but only tend to trust facility-level statements. Generic warnings like "may contain peanuts" could mean a range of things and are just not specific enough for me to risk eating.

Step 3: Search for Additional Allergen Information Online

If there is no PAL facility-level statement on the packaging and the product doesn't list my allergen in the ingredients, I'll check the brand's website for an FAQ section or any allergen information from my phone while in the store. This information can be difficult to find and may not be immediately visible in the website's navigation bar or even available at all. In those cases, I'll search online with terms like "[brand name] + [allergen]" to locate relevant details, which might appear under sections like Nutrition or News. However, brands don't always provide allergen details online, and checking for a date is also useful to ensure the information isn't outdated.

If the information isn't available on the packaging or website and I still want to determine if the product is safe, I'll email the company. I will usually reach out about all their products, but sometimes, I'll make it specific about a single product if that's all

I'm interested in. Here's a baseline template you can personalize as needed:

> *Hello, I'm interested in purchasing your products and need to know if they are safe for my anaphylactic peanut allergy. To limit cross-contact risk, I avoid products made in facilities where peanut ingredients, such as peanuts, peanut oil, peanut butter, or peanut flour, are used. Could you please tell me if any peanut ingredients are used in your facilities? I appreciate the information. Thank you!*

If they reply, I can ask further questions if their initial response isn't detailed enough. If finding a specific safe product is too challenging, I often adapt by substituting ingredients with safer options I already have or by ordering something similar from allergen-safe brands.

For me, grocery shopping usually means visiting multiple stores to gather all the ingredients I need, as much of what's on the shelves either lacks clear labeling or isn't safe. This flexibility to shop around and seek alternatives is a privilege—not everyone has the option to shop at multiple places or buy specialty items online, and many must rely on whatever is available at their nearest store.

To prevent wasting money on food or making returns, I often take photos of barcodes while shopping and email the manufacturers once I get home. Later, I buy only the products that have confirmed they don't process peanuts in their facility. I also send follow-up emails periodically for items that last a while, just to check if anything has changed before buying them again.

Some of my friends and family have started helping me with this task when I need them to, such as around a busy holiday. There are also Facebook resource groups, blogs, and loads of online forums that post product brand leads for helpful allergen information that isn't always provided willingly by companies. Having a lead on a company or brand that labels their products clearly can make finding a facility without your allergens much more efficient than contacting brands at random.

I've also learned that reaching out to a brand can have a bigger impact than just getting an answer to an allergy question. Emailing manufacturers to share how much you love and rely on their safe products not only reinforces the demand but can encourage them to maintain allergen-safe practices. Sometimes they even send coupons or special offers. You can also contact the grocery stores you shop at to request they carry these products, helping ensure they remain accessible to the broader community.

These strategies help throughout the year, but certain times, like holidays, can be especially challenging for managing food allergies. Beyond the extra planning and vigilance needed with treats and food everywhere, there's also the creeping feeling of exclusion when so many celebrations revolve around eating together. Thankfully, as allergy awareness has grown, it's starting to influence the holidays, too.

The Teal Pumpkin is now widely recognized by major retailers as the symbol for food allergy awareness, which is an exciting development for Halloween, a time so focused on candy. It encourages non-food treats as valid options, making celebrations safer and less food-focused. If you haven't heard of the Teal Pumpkin Project, check out their website and be sure to add your house to their map each year if you plan to give out non-food treats.

Making Halloween inclusive in this way goes beyond food allergies. Consider children with celiac disease, diabetes, tube-feeding needs, or other dietary restrictions. In fact, I learned many ways to additionally be inclusive around Halloween from the nonprofit Never Give Up which got me thinking about creating an accessible pathway for trick-or-treaters, considering mobility challenges, fine motor skills, and sensory sensitivities.

They explain how non-food alternatives like glow sticks, small toys, or placing treats in easy-to-open bags can make a big difference. Celebrating inclusively also means respecting that not every child will speak, wear a costume, or participate in traditional trick-or-treating for developmental,cultural, or personal reasons. Some children may be older but still enjoy the fun of Halloween, and they focus on creating thoughtful, accessible, and allergy-aware spaces so everyone can participate safely and joyfully.

Tried-and-True Strategies for Safer Food Shopping

Reading food labels can sometimes feel like navigating a maze of fine print, especially depending on your allergies. However, a few strategic approaches can make it far more manageable. Here are my top three tips to help simplify the process and find safe options without getting bogged down by details:

Find Reliable Brands & Stick to Them

Identifying trustworthy brands that clearly communicate allergens can significantly simplify your shopping experience. As you explore various products, you'll find which brands consistently provide helpful allergen information on their websites, packaging, or through direct email discussions.

While this process may feel like a massive undertaking, building a list of reliable products will make it easier over time. Although it's imperative to verify ingredient statements with each purchase (as they can change), having a go-to list of trusted brands will streamline your shopping and make it easier for anyone shopping on your behalf.

Be Mindful of Contaminated Produce

I always wash my produce before eating, but ideally, I also try to wash all produce thoroughly before putting it away and again before eating it. This limits the contamination of my home in the interim between buying and eating it.

It might sound extreme initially, but I also pay close attention to where certain produce is grown if I can easily find the information. For example, I exercise extra caution with Georgia, Florida, or Alabama items, as my allergen (peanuts) may share land or equipment with these crops. While I try not to stress about this, it's worth keeping in the back of your mind based on the specific allergies you manage. This awareness can be helpful in the rare event that a reaction occurs and you're unsure of the cause.

I don't usually focus on farm and garden companion plants, but I've learned that peanuts share similar growing conditions with vegetables like carrots, squash, tomatoes, cucumbers, and potatoes. Because of my peanut allergy, I carefully wash these items along with peaches which are often grown on the same farms as peanuts and pecans. Whenever possible, I prefer to buy produce from regions like California, where my allergen is not commonly grown.

Adopting a contamination mindset means recognizing that contamination can happen at any stage—from transit and grocery store handling to checkout and preparation of ingredients in a contaminated environment. In case you skipped around while reading, for more details on cross-contact, see Chapter 3.

Use the Trader Joe's Phone Line

As a grocery store, Trader Joe's stands out for offering a free phone line during weekday store hours to provide allergen information and answer related questions. This service has been invaluable for me, and I highly recommend it if you have a TJs nearby. However, it would be even better if they extended this service to weekends and included current allergen information directly on their product labels, so consumers wouldn't need to call each time.

Regardless, I greatly appreciate their current process, as it's better than no allergen communication with consumers. I've always made the calls myself, although I've heard some people in the food allergy community have asked in-store customer service employees to assist.

Their product phone line as of publishing is 626-599-3817.

Additional Labeling Law Information

Up until recently, the FDA's *Food Labeling Guide* served as a comprehensive resource detailing food labeling requirements. However, this guide has since been removed from the FDA's website.

For the most up-to-date information on food labeling laws and regulations, you can visit the FDA's Labeling & Nutrition Guidance Documents page. This section includes the latest guidance documents, proposed rules, and updates on nutrition labeling requirements.

The National Agricultural Law Center's Food Labeling Overview, found on their website, summarizes US food labeling laws and key legislation, including the Nutrition Labeling and Education Act (NLEA) and the Food Allergen Labeling and Consumer Protection Act (FALCPA).

FALCPA requires that the top food allergens—milk, eggs, fish, crustacean shellfish, tree nuts, peanuts, wheat, and soy—be clearly identified on food labels to protect consumers. In 2023, the FASTER Act added sesame as the ninth major allergen, updating labeling requirements to include sesame as well. Along with the FDA's website, this resource helps consumers understand US food labeling laws and interpret labels accurately to make informed choices.

A Vision for Better Food Labeling

Throughout this book, I've highlighted the urgent need for stricter food manufacturing regulations in the US. I've been greatly inspired by the EU's labeling standards, which I've experienced firsthand during travel, as well as reading about Australia's Allergen

Bureau's VITAL program and South Korea's labeling standards. The US has the ability to create a system tailored to our unique needs that aligns with what the food allergy community finds most useful. While changes to labeling laws require a substantial shift for US food manufacturers, they're necessary for consumer safety—and ultimately, without consumers, their products don't sell.

Here's a quick overview of food labeling laws in the European Union (EU), Canada, Australia, and South Korea, showcasing their key requirements and differences. While the legislative process is often slow and uncertain, data-driven advocacy can create lasting improvements for consumers with dietary restrictions and food manufacturers. A recurring fear within the food allergy community is manufacturer backlash—something that's happened in the past when new standards were introduced. Instead of following them to help consumers, they added the allergens to more products and eliminated PALs.

To mitigate this, advocates with legislative experience and beyond are working to gain manufacturers' buy-in upfront and craft policies they'd be more willing to implement. This collaborative approach aims to reduce friction and avoid the added stress of potential pushback.

Comparing Global Labeling: EU, CA, ROK, & AU

Looking at food labeling systems established in the European Union, Canada, South Korea, and Australia side-by-side helps to see their strategies for allergen labeling, allergen management, and nutritional information.

- Scope: The European Union (EU) and Canadian (CA) regulations encompass comprehensive food labeling requirements, while South Korea (Republic of Korea, or ROK) mandates both allergen disclosures and Precautionary Allergen Labeling (PAL) for shared manufacturing environments.

Australia's VITAL program, on the other hand, focuses primarily on managing allergen cross-contact.

- Mandatory vs. Voluntary: The EU, CA, and ROK require mandatory allergen labeling.
- ROK specifically mandates a distinct warning if a manufacturing process handles allergenic and non-allergenic products, advising consumers of the potential for cross-contact. Australia's VITAL program remains voluntary but is widely adopted as a best practice in the industry.
- Allergen Management: All these systems emphasize allergen transparency. ROK requires labeling for 22 priority allergens, including shellfish, pine nuts, and peaches, and additional labeling measures for potential cross-contact. Australia's VITAL program allows for structured cross-contact risk assessment, focusing on clear, data-backed allergen disclosures.
- Nutritional Information: The EU and CA require nutritional details, while ROK mandates them specifically for processed foods. Australia's VITAL program excludes this, as its primary focus is allergen cross-contact.

So there you have it—exciting opportunities for US labeling laws await! We're uniquely positioned at an advantage to not have to start from scratch and be able to develop a food labeling standard that merges the best elements from these international systems.

Integrating mandatory allergen transparency like that of the EU, Canada, and ROK could improve labeling practices. ROK stands out as the only country, to my knowledge, that mandates some level of Precautionary Allergen Labeling (PAL) for potential cross-contact. The US can create a robust framework that ensures consumer safety and effectively addresses allergen cross-contact. Embracing such a standard would align us with global best practices and greatly enhance consumer protection and information.

It's worth noting that these countries also have universal healthcare systems, which inherently prioritize public health and safety. Their approaches ensure that quality healthcare, including robust food safety and labeling practices, is accessible and affordable—or even free—for their citizens. This stands in stark contrast to the United States, where the lack of universal healthcare creates disparities in health outcomes and limits access to essential services. As the US seeks to advance labeling standards, it must also address the broader systemic issue of equitable healthcare access to truly support the well-being of its population.

Right now feels like a critical moment for US healthcare to change to help the majority of people. In July 2025, the "One Big Beautiful Bill Act" was signed into law, which includes nearly $1 trillion in Medicaid cuts over the next decade. The United States spends far more on healthcare than other wealthy countries, yet life expectancy remains lower than in countries that provide universal coverage. In short, the for-profit system we are accustomed to isn't working for the people it's supposed to serve.

Thom Hartmann's 2021 book, *The Hidden History of American Healthcare: Why Sickness Bankrupts You and Makes Others Insanely Rich*, explains in an easy-to-read format how the US model relies on private insurance in ways that other industrialized nations do not, highlighting both the inequities and the missed opportunities for reform.

I hope we can use this moment of crisis as a wake-up call to completely rethink healthcare, moving toward a system that guarantees care for all, because healthcare is not a privilege; it is a human right. Every person, regardless of income or circumstance, deserves access to the care they need to live a healthy, dignified life. I do not believe in a system that prioritizes billionaires over the health and well-being of the public. Wealth at that scale comes from somewhere, and too often it is extracted at the expense of other people's lives, safety, and access to basic necessities like healthcare. True justice in healthcare means ensuring that no one is left behind for the sake of profit or extreme wealth accumulation.

The Case of the Misleading Yogurt

This section delves into a specific example from a blog article on my website about misleading labels, highlighting a significant flaw in current labeling regulations and the everyday risks they pose.

It all started during a trip to my local grocery store, where I was on a mission to find a safe yogurt. Yogurt has always been a rare treat, since most brands don't clearly state whether they share facilities with peanuts. I often must contact manufacturers directly, which leads to a mixed bag of responses—sometimes I get clear and helpful information, other times the answers are vague or unhelpful; and occasionally, I don't hear back at all. This frustrating process highlights a major gap in labeling practices that affects many consumers like me.

This particular time, I spotted a yogurt with a large "nut-free" logo on the front label—"Score!" I thought. But then I flipped to the back ingredients panel and saw, "Made in a facility that contains nuts." *Huh?* Maybe I misread the nut-free logo. I flipped it back over and stared at it—nope, I read it right the first time. I let out an audible *ugh*.

This troubling discrepancy left me questioning what types of nuts are used and feeling uneasy about the product's safety for those with life-threatening nut allergies, despite the nut-free marketing proudly displayed on the front.

Fortunately, I caught this conflicting information before actually eating the product. Had I relied solely on the front nut-free claim, I could have put my life in danger. This experience shows why reviewing labels is essential, as our current labeling laws can sometimes be misleading. A good practice is to check ingredient labels three times: once at the store, again when putting items away at home, and one last time before eating. This approach increases your chances of catching discrepancies or errors—after all, everyone makes mistakes. In the food allergy community, a single mistake can carry the weight of a life-threatening consequence.

While this instance may seem minor, it represents a recurring problem across countless brands. This example illustrates how confusing and misleading information can arise frequently. It underscores the urgent need for the US to adopt consistent, standardized verbiage on ingredient panels.

Imagine if every product included standardized verbiage detailing its ingredients and a reliable allergen statement, such as, "Produced in a facility with tree nuts, peanuts, soy, and wheat." Such a standard would make it easier for consumers to understand potential cross-contact risks for the top 9 allergens. Without this level of transparency, consumers are left guessing—and for those of us with life-threatening food allergies, that's a dangerous gamble.

Additionally, stricter regulations are needed for front-of-packaging marketing to prevent misleading claims like "nut-free" unless these terms are clearly defined. Standardization is crucial so that claims have specific and consistent meanings, such as "no nuts are present in the facility." Currently, such claims can be harmful, particularly for individuals with IgE-mediated allergies, who can experience anaphylaxis from even trace amounts of an allergen.

Accurate labeling of the top 9 allergens, as well as all ingredients—is not just a matter of convenience; it's essential for consumer safety. And let's not forget: this discussion doesn't even touch on allergens beyond the top 9—an entirely different and equally important issue that still needs attention.

The reality is that 170+ foods have been reported to cause allergic reactions. While labeling for the top 9 is a critical step forward, it cannot be the only long-term solution for the food allergy community. Allergens outside of the top 9, many of which can also trigger anaphylaxis, are especially difficult to manage since they aren't required to be explicitly listed on ingredient labels or disclosed in facility-level statements. If you've ever had to avoid allergens beyond the top 9, you already know how frustrating it is to decode ambiguous terms like "natural spices" and "natural flavoring" on ingredient panels.

I don't claim to have all the solutions—not by a long shot. My goal is to raise awareness and help pave the way for positive changes in the community. Starting with the top 9 allergens is a necessary and impactful step that will benefit many people, but it is only the beginning. We must continue to push for transparency from food manufacturers. There is still much work to be done to ensure everyone can make safe and informed eating choices.

The 2017 Clif Bar Recall

In 2017, Clif Bars and Clif Kid ZBars issued a voluntary recall due to potential allergen contamination. It was for their Chocolate Mint flavor, as well as Clif Kid Zbar Protein Chocolate Mint and Chocolate Chip flavors, due to the possible presence of undeclared peanuts and tree nuts, including almonds, Brazil nuts, cashews, hazelnuts, macadamia nuts, pecans, walnuts, and coconuts. This incident made me more aware of the risks associated with product recalls and reinforced my decision to avoid products from facilities that process my allergens.

By the time of this recall in 2017, I had been several years removed from my anaphylactic experience at the allergist's office. As described earlier in this chapter, I had already developed my method for avoiding products from facilities that used peanuts. Although adopting this practice required an initial mental and time investment, it has dramatically improved my quality of life. Avoiding these products has now become second nature, making it easier for me to manage my allergies effectively.

In my late teens and early 20s, Clif Bars, Luna Bars, and

Quest Protein Bars were my go-to breakfasts as I rushed to work or college classes. Back then, I was unaware of the significant gaps in food labeling laws and protections. Due to this, I was unknowingly consuming multiple items daily that were made in facilities that also processed peanuts, often on shared equipment. This lack of knowledge led to frequent cross-contact allergic reactions, leaving me baffled and frustrated, as the ingredient lists showed no mention of peanuts.

Even after learning about these gaps in 2013-2014, it took me years to adjust my habits and find the willpower to eliminate potentially unsafe products that were convenient and much less expensive than most allergy-safe options. By the time the recall occurred in 2017, I was already avoiding foods labeled "may contain" peanuts. This was fortunate, since my favorite Clif Bar flavor had just been voluntarily recalled for potential undisclosed peanuts.

Although I wasn't personally affected by the recall, it was terrifying. It underscored how many people unknowingly consume unsafe products because of gaps in food labeling laws. The

The constant and harsh reality is the fear of encountering an allergen in a product that has yet to be recalled. Despite our best efforts to stay vigilant, it can lead to allergic reactions with potentially fatal outcomes.

This recall starkly underscores the limitations of relying solely on food allergy vigilance, highlighting the urgent need for a more robust food labeling system. No matter how careful you are, recalls can still occur. For those of us with food allergies, this situation amplifies the need for cautious practices and strengthens the call for advocacy and awareness in the food allergy community. Until improved food practices are established by manufacturers, recalls serve as a stark reminder of the constant risks we face.

The Grain Craft Flour Recall: A Widespread Contamination

If you were managing a life-threatening allergy in the US in 2016, you likely remember the nationwide Grain Craft flour contamination headlines. While detailed articles on the incident are available online, I'll provide a brief synopsis and explain why grasping the implications of this event is crucial. This contamination event is noteworthy because it accentuates the significant risks of inadequate allergen labeling and cross-contact management. It underscores the need for more rigorous food safety practices and demonstrates the challenges individuals with food allergies face when manufacturers fail to prevent or adequately disclose potential allergen contamination.

In 2016, Grain Craft, a large flour supplier, discovered that its wheat flour was contaminated with peanut residue. This was particularly alarming because the tainted flour had been distributed to hundreds of other suppliers, which then passed the flour further down the chain to their own nested brands and companies. As a result, the contamination spread widely, affecting a diverse range of products. Ultimately, it impacted baked goods and restaurant meals and even made its way into pre-prepared and packaged frozen foods.

To provide some name-brand examples, the contaminated flour found its way into products like Cinnabon Stix, Hostess snack cakes, and Chick-fil-A chocolate chunk cookies. The risk of exposure for people with peanut allergies was too extensive and impossible to fully gauge.

As someone with a peanut allergy, this meant that even foods I typically considered "safe," with a straightforward ingredients label, could have been jeopardized by this recall. The widespread distribution of the contaminated flour heightened the risk of accidental exposure, creating a daunting challenge for individuals trying to avoid potential allergic reactions.

The scale of this incident, along with others discussed in this book, further magnifies the need for stricter food safety practices and more thorough monitoring. It illuminates the critical necessity for effective measures to prevent cross-contact with undisclosed ingredients and to detect recalls before they reach consumers. Particularly when dealing with recalls on such a large scale, I was driven to eat more cleanly to avoid processed products, as my trust in food brands was severely shaken.

Consumers eventually learned that the cross-contact happened during the farm's milling process, causing peanut particles to get mixed with the wheat. It is suspected that the contamination might have occurred at one point when the red wheat and peanuts were processed or stored together, either in shared facilities or during transport. The FDA investigated this incident to try and pinpoint the source, but despite extensive analysis, the exact source of the contamination was never determined. The only thing they knew for sure was that peanut ingredients were present. It still unsettles me that both Grain Craft and the FDA were unable to identify the definitive source during their inspections of the milling facilities, even after testing the flour samples.

This situation exposes further vulnerabilities in our food safety system, especially in handling and processing ingredients at their source and in their raw state. Despite my current "method" of inquiring about allergens in the facilities where products are made, these efforts would not have prevented an allergic reaction. The contamination originated from the raw materials themselves, which were compromised before reaching the manufacturing stage.

Addressing these challenges, from farm to final product, requires a concerted effort to mandate and implement stricter regulations and enhanced monitoring practices for each ingredient. By strengthening these measures, food manufacturers can better mitigate cross-contact risks and improve food products' safety nationwide. For more detailed information on this particular recall, you can refer to the original 2016 articles in *Food Safety News* and *Foods for Better Health*.

Closing Thoughts & Additional Context

- Understanding Label Limitations: Food labeling in the US is complex and often inconsistent. While the FDA requires clear, standardized labeling for the top 9 allergens—except when they're present in highly refined oils—product recalls still happen. There is currently no requirement for transparency around shared equipment, facility-level cross-contact, or allergens outside the top 9. This leaves many consumers, especially those with less common food allergies, in a constant state of uncertainty. Advocacy groups are working hard to change this, but we need broader public awareness and support to pressure food manufacturers and regulators to take these gaps seriously.

- Angioedema and "Anaphylaxis of the Stomach": A nurse at my allergist's office once shared that *angioedema* (facial swelling reactions that can still require epinephrine even without throat involvement) and *gastrointestinal anaphylaxis* (sometimes called "anaphylaxis of the stomach," which can also require epinephrine but is less understood in terms of whether it can be fatal) are both important to know about and worth further research, since broadening our understanding of these reactions can improve recognition, treatment, and ultimately patient safety. The 2023 guidelines from AAAAI and ACAAI recommend epinephrine as the first-line treatment, because less-typical symptoms can escalate or occur alongside hidden systemic effects. The uncertainty lies more in the fatality risk of GI-only anaphylaxis, since the data is limited, but the medical standard remains: when in doubt, Epi first.

- Regulation Gaps: Precautionary Allergen Labeling (PAL)

statements like "may contain" and "nut-free" or "made in a facility with…" are unregulated and not verified as being accurate, so approach them with caution. This highlights the need for more rigorous food labeling laws, including front-of-label packaging.

- Wheat vs. Gluten: A Labeling Gap: In the US, wheat is one of the top 9 allergens and must be clearly disclosed on food labels. Gluten, however, is not, so manufacturers are not required to list it, even though it's the protein in wheat that causes reactions for many people. This distinction can be confusing, especially for those avoiding gluten for health reasons or managing wheat allergies. People also need to be aware of products made with modified wheat flour, which can be technically gluten-free but still contain wheat protein. So, a product labeled "gluten-free" does not automatically mean it is free of wheat, and vice versa, making it challenging to navigate ingredient lists safely. To address this gap, a citizen petition was started by Celiac Journey, founded by Jon, Leslie, Lexi, and Jax Bari from Philadelphia, which provides a platform to support the petition, advocate for change, and work to get gluten named as a major food allergen in the US—as it already is in Europe and Canada.

- The Allergen Disclosure in Non-food Articles (ADINA) Act: This proposed legislation aims to extend allergen labeling requirements for the top 9 allergens and gluten-containing grains to medications, including both over the counter and prescription drugs. This is an essential development because current laws do not mandate such labeling for medications, and pharmacists and doctors often lack a quick way to access this critical information. Contact your representatives about supporting this act, and check their website to learn more: www.adinaact.com

- Tracking Legislation at Federal and State Levels: If you're interested in tracking acts and bills in Congress, I often use the website Congress.gov. It's an excellent resource for finding out about introduced acts and passed bills and learning about your congressional representatives and what they're supporting. I have used the site while lobbying for food allergy policies and to review the types of bills my state representatives have previously supported. This helps me tailor my approach to be more emotionally and persuasively resonant. The website lets users check if representatives co-sponsor any of the federal bills they've asked them to support and allows users to flag bills to "watch" and receive email alerts. I highly recommend it. Surprisingly, I was introduced to Congress.gov by a fellow passenger on my flight home from D.C. after one of FARE's previous Courage at Congress events. He was a veteran in his 70s lobbying for veterans' rights, and I was so impressed by him. Not only did he teach me how to use the Congress website, but he also asked me a couple genuine questions about my food allergy to understand it better, first asking if it was okay for him to ask me the questions and making sure nothing he ate on the flight would impact me negatively.

- Personal Food Labeling Strategy: Navigating food choices with food allergies means making educated guesses and taking calculated risks, especially when allergen information is unclear. To eat more safely, you can develop a personalized method for reading food labels tailored to your unique needs and allergies. This process typically includes examining ingredient lists carefully, checking for facility-level allergen statements about what allergens are in the facility or on shared equipment, and searching online for additional allergen information and/or contacting companies directly to ask about allergens being in products, in the same facility, or on shared equipment.

- Importance of Reliable Brands: On my website, I keep a detailed document listing trusted food brands that usually provide clear allergen information. I created this resource not only as a personal reference—because there's so much information to remember, and I inevitably forget which brands I've found safe—but also so my friends and family can use it to find potential safe options. While each product still needs to be checked carefully since ingredients can change, having this list helps streamline the shopping process and reduces the risk of accidental exposure. Building and maintaining a list of reliable brands for yourself and your friends and family can be an important step toward making everyday food choices safer and less stressful for those managing food allergies.

- Dining Out: When dining out at a restaurant or bakery, obtaining detailed information about individual ingredients and their facilities is challenging, so I tend to limit eating out. This precaution has significantly reduced the number of reactions I experience. However, when I do decide to eat out, the process I follow is that I email the establishment in advance to address any concerns and discuss the use of peanuts or peanut-derived ingredients in the kitchen or bar, such as peanut oil or peanut flour. I also ask whether the kitchen is shared, used as a co-op kitchen, or involved in catering, as this can introduce allergens into the space they may not initially consider. For places I visit regularly and where I've had positive experiences, I typically send follow-up emails every few months to check for any changes and then verify with the staff in person once I'm there. I've found that when I don't do this, I start having more allergic reactions, which is why I continue with this practice. I try not to waiver on my emailing process, and I'll explain why with a couple of stories. I had called a local pizza pub to ask about their kitchen, and they assured me that they didn't use peanuts on the menu over the phone. I still emailed, and only after that did I learn that while peanuts weren't used in their food, the bar served a house-made peanut butter tequila shot prepared in the kitchen, which could easily introduce kitchen cross-contact exposure. Another instance, which my friend still references in shock, happened while traveling. I had emailed ahead and found a food truck that was nut-free and had good allergen protocols. After eating there, my friend wanted to advocate and help me find a sweet treat, and I explained my emailing process but let her ask around to the nearby trucks if she wanted. She eagerly inquired about allergens to another food truck and was told, "no peanuts at all!" We thought we were safe, but as she looked at the menu more closely in line, she noticed a peanut butter smoothie listed. Both the manager and her had initially missed it, and she was horrified that she nearly influenced me to bend my rule. She kindly but firmly pointed it out to the staff, who acknowledged their oversight.

- Setting a Precedent for Safer Dining: These experiences are why I find so much value in emailing ahead. There is no perfect system beyond trying to push for mandatory menu transparency laws like California's ADDE Act (SB 68), which provides accountability and repercussions. California's new law is paving the way for similar measures in other states and at the federal level. Just as California led the nation decades ago by pioneering nutrition labeling—which eventually became a nationwide standard—this bill now sparks similar progress in allergen disclosure. By requiring the top 9 allergens to be clearly listed on menus, it sets a new precedent. And while it doesn't eliminate risk or address cross-contact, it underscores the same principles that shaped the EU's allergen laws: clarity, safety, awareness, and accessibility for consumers.

7

NAVIGATING CROSS-CONTACT

Practical Strategies

Throughout this book, I've shared my journey with food allergies, beginning in infancy when my family managed them and continuing through childhood, adolescence, and now, as an adult, managing my peanut allergy independently. I describe myself as airborne and cross-contact allergic, and even with my extensive allergy experience, I'm always discovering new ways cross-contact can happen.

This section shares practical steps for detecting and preventing cross-contact, an issue often underdiscussed despite its seriousness. While this chapter may feel more technical or dry, the steps I outline, from understanding cross-contact nuances to implementing helpful protocols and staying vigilant while out and about, are designed to protect those navigating the complexities of food allergies.

As with all the advice in this book, these steps are flexible and should be tailored to your needs and preferences. Given the nearly endless ways cross-contact can occur, this list cannot cover every potential instance—though I wish it could! The reality is that new factors continue to emerge as the world evolves.

Building Cross-Contact Awareness: A 3-Step Guide

Step 1: Defining Cross-Contact

- *What is cross-contact?* Cross-contact, commonly known as CC, refers to the unintentional transfer of allergens from one food to another. Even minimal contact can cause an allergic reaction.

- *What is the difference between cross-contact and cross-contamination?* Cross-contact involves the transfer of allergens, while cross-contamination typically refers to the transfer of harmful bacteria or pathogens from one surface or food to another. This highlights the distinction between allergen protein exposure and microbial contamination.

- *Will using hand sanitizer remove "cross-contact" of allergen proteins?* No. Hand sanitizer effectively kills germs and bacteria but does not remove allergen proteins responsible for cross-contact. Similarly, while a wet wipe may help remove residue, it may not eliminate all allergen proteins. Thorough washing with soap and water is the most reliable method to effectively remove allergen proteins. However, wet wipes can be useful for surface cleaning and are convenient when soap and water aren't an option.

Step 2: Practicing Identifying Cross-Contact

Cultivating cross-contact awareness is a skill that improves with practice. In this section, I'll explore various settings where cross-contact can occur, helping you develop a keen eye for potential risks. By consistently paying attention to trace amounts of allergens, you can more effectively identify and prevent cross-contact.

- Cross-contact is an ongoing challenge if you're allergic to trace amounts of your allergens. However, it can be successfully managed in many situations with minimal effort, hopefully leading to much less food allergy fear and anxiety.

- Increasing Observation and Awareness: Consider common areas where cross-contact might occur, such as home kitchens, restaurant kitchens, food delivery services, cafeterias, and food product manufacturing facilities. In restaurants, cross-contact can happen through shared cooking surfaces and utensils or when employees bring allergens from outside environments. In food manufacturing facilities, cross-contact can occur during production, processing, and packaging.

- Look for Environmental Examples: Expand your awareness to specific environments like homes, stores, schools, healthcare facilities, gyms, outdoor events such as festivals and parks, and other public areas such as community centers and libraries.
- Real-Life Scenarios: Consider how cross-contact can occur in the above settings. For example, community centers often host events with food, increasing the risk of cross-contact for individuals with food allergies. Attendees could communicate their dietary needs to event organizers and inquire about the types of foods present or that may have been present, to assess risk and comfort level before going. Similarly, picnic areas and park playgrounds can pose risks due to shared spaces like picnic tables, grilling areas, and playground equipment. These surfaces are often not cleaned regularly, so individuals with food allergies should be cautious in order to minimize the risk of allergen exposure in these public settings.
- Improvement Over Time: Be patient with yourself as you work on honing this cross-contact identifying skill. While understanding and managing cross-contact risk can significantly reduce the frequency of allergic reactions, it's necessary to acknowledge that cross-contact may still occur despite your best efforts. This is a challenging reality of living with food allergies. However, with continued practice and experience, you'll become more skilled at identifying and managing these risks, leading to better protection and hopefully fewer allergic reactions.

Step 3: Defining Your Cross-Contact Boundaries

The final step in managing cross-contact is clearly defining your own personal boundaries for handling it. If you're assisting someone with a food allergy, it's essential to understand and respect their specific boundaries. While aware of my limits, I make it a point to ask others about their comfort level with trace amounts of their allergen. I recognize that reactions to cross-contact can vary—some may not worry about it, while others must be constantly vigilant.

Setting and communicating clear boundaries isn't just a food allergy management skill—it's a fundamental life skill that promotes healthy relationships, emotional well-being, and personal growth. Establishing clear cross-contact boundaries can be incredibly empowering for those with food allergies. Beyond ensuring safety, these boundaries support self-care by helping individuals manage stress and prioritize their needs. They foster mutual respect and trust in relationships, improve communication, and enhance understanding. Well-defined boundaries also build confidence and assertiveness, promoting a balanced approach to personal and interpersonal needs and contributing to overall well-being.

I've sometimes felt like a burden because of my allergy. However, as I practiced communicating my boundaries, I felt more secure in my assertiveness and less like a bother. I remind myself that anyone can develop a food allergy or disability at any time and that my needs are deserving of acceptance and respect.

To help overcome this lingering sense of being a burden, I turn to this visualization:

Close your eyes and take a deep breath. Picture someone you care about—someone you naturally want to protect and support—needing the same accommodations or care that you require. Notice how effortlessly you advocate for them, how naturally you honor their needs without judgment. Now, gently imagine the roles reversed: you in their place, and them in yours. Feel the same compassion, certainty, and care you extended to them flowing toward yourself. Allow yourself to validate your own needs with the kindness and confidence you so readily give to others.

Protecting Yourself Through Clear Boundaries:

Understanding and effectively communicating your limits allows you to navigate various settings with greater confidence and safety. Here are some practical tips to help you define and enforce your cross-contact boundaries:

Tip 1: Personal Boundaries

Evaluate your comfort level with potential cross-contact situations based on your allergy history. If it helps, take a moment to journal about this, reflecting on your ideal situation with managing cross-contact to limit allergic reactions.

- Real-Life Example: If you have a peanut allergy, you may avoid events where peanuts are served. Communicate this decision to friends and event hosts to ensure your safety. If they cannot accommodate your needs, explain your reason for not attending, as this helps others understand the risk and raises awareness about food allergy severity.

Tip 2: Preventative Measures

Establish your preferred strategies to prevent cross-contact. These might include bringing utensils, avoiding certain foods or locations, bringing wet wipes to clean shared surfaces and clearly communicating your accommodations to others.

- Real-Life Example: When dining out and planning to get a salad with a cross-contact allergy to tree nuts and peanuts, consider bringing your own toppings if you're concerned about cross-contact. For instance, if a salad contains dried cherries and olives—bulk ingredients often processed on equipment shared with nuts—you might prefer to avoid those toppings. Instead, bring a small container or baggie with your safe alternatives and explain your choices to your server, requesting that the salad be served without those risky toppings. Additionally, you can ask the restaurant about their procedures for preventing cross-contact and inquire about their ingredient sourcing to ensure your safety. I suggest confirming this information via email before your visit in order to have evidence in writing.

Tip 3: Communication

Mastering the art of communicating your boundaries and needs is something I consider a high priority, though it can take time. Whether at home, in social settings, or in public spaces, finding a communication method that feels authentic to you can be powerful. This ensures you can express yourself clearly and confidently. I've discovered it's much easier to speak my way, using language and approaches that feel true to who I am.

- Real-Life Example: At a family gathering, clearly express your allergy concerns by requesting that certain foods be kept separate or fully eliminated. You might say, "I have an anaphylactic dairy allergy, so please keep all dishes containing dairy on a separate table and use different serving utensils." Or "I have an anaphylactic dairy allergy, and I'll only be able to attend if no dairy is used while I'm there." Whatever your boundary is, this approach ensures that your needs are clearly understood and helps create a safer environment.

By setting and regularly enforcing food allergy boundaries, you protect yourself from allergens and help educate those around you. Consistently communicating your needs fosters a more aware and considerate community, benefiting everyone. One of my boundaries is not working in environments where peanuts are consumed. This is because I am not only cross-contact but also airborne allergic to peanut particles. I was tired of regularly having to leave work and use sick time, PTO, or unpaid leave due to allergic reactions.

Plus, constantly monitoring for reactions was stressful since the likelihood was fairly high. I established this based on my health needs, which multiple employers have respected and successfully upheld. Seeing others willingly accommodate and respect my allergy boundaries has boosted my self-confidence and reassured me that asking for my food allergy needs to be met is reasonable and deserved.

Real-World Examples and Context

For those interested in a more detailed exploration of cross-contact, this section offers in-depth examples of potential allergen exposure in settings such as homes and stores that we encounter daily in the world around us.

Homes

Cross-contact risks can arise in home environments, even with careful allergen avoidance. For instance, visitors who may carry them on their clothes or personal items can introduce trace amounts of allergens. Imagine someone recently at a restaurant that uses your allergens or walking in a space with your allergens on the ground. Pets can also carry allergens on their fur or in their saliva, so it's helpful to ask about their contamination level if they're visiting.

Allergen proteins can linger on contaminated items brought inside, so it's advantageous to remain aware of these potential risks. While it's challenging and likely impossible to completely eliminate all cross-contact, staying vigilant, asking questions, and trusting your instincts can help manage them effectively. This approach can reduce stress and help create a safer environment for everyone.

Grocery Stores and Retail Environments

Stores that offer a wide range of food products, such as grocery stores, convenience stores, and gas stations, can present increased cross-contact risks due to the concentration of various food allergens in one place. Common areas to be aware of include check-out lane conveyor belts and bulk sections where items may be without packaging.

You might find labeled allergen-free items with sticky, contaminated packaging at the grocery store. Similarly, many people touch the check-out payment pad, which may be cleaned infrequently. Staying aware of these potential risks and taking precautions, like using hand wipes after shopping or wiping down items before putting them away at home, can help manage exposure.

Pet Stores and Clinics

Pet stores and veterinary clinics can pose cross-contact risks due to the high level of allergens. Dust from pet foods containing allergens like peanuts, wheat, tree nuts, and dairy can become airborne in these environments. Allergens may also be present in pet products, on pets, and in their saliva. For example, I've encountered peanuts in pet stores and clinics through birdseed and dog treats. To reduce the risk of allergic reactions, it's important to stay vigilant and take precautions, such as wearing a mask in areas with high dust levels and immediately washing any contaminated clothes upon returning home. If you have someone else who can shop for you in pet stores or other areas where your allergens are prevalent and out in the open, that's an option, too!

Educational Institutions

Schools, colleges, and other educational settings can pose cross-contact risks due to high foot traffic and shared spaces. Risks arise when individuals bring outside food into these environments or when cafeteria meals and vending machine items often contain common allergens. People eating at desks can unintentionally contaminate shared areas like chairs, door handles, and desks. I worked with the HR department at my college to draft a disability letter for my food allergy, which I provided to my professors. The letter, signed by the college, required that they make an announcement and hang signs on my classroom doors prohibiting peanut products in my classes. While this didn't guarantee that rooms would be free of other allergens from different classes, it ensured that no one in my vicinity was consuming peanuts. I'd often use wet wipes to clean surfaces off before touching them, like my seat and desk, in these settings.

Now You've Got the Mindset

By adopting a high-level perspective on cross-contact and focusing on overarching themes of risk mitigation, individuals managing food allergies can navigate various environments more confidently and reduce the likelihood of allergic reactions. Although specific examples are helpful, they can only cover some possible cross-contact scenarios due to the endless range of potential exposures. Therefore, developing a cross-contact mindset is essential for identifying and addressing situations where cross-contact may occur and taking proactive steps to minimize risks effectively.

Staying Empowered in Cross-Contact Management

Addressing the specific ways allergen cross-contact can occur is deeply healing for me, as managing cross-contact is one of the most challenging aspects of living with my anaphylactic allergy. Despite extensive searching, I am still looking for resources from doctors or allergists online that thoroughly explore developing a cross-contact mindset like mine here. Perhaps such content exists, and I've yet to come across it, but this chapter serves as the resource I wish I could have relied on in the past.

In detailing this, I discovered it was more challenging

than anticipated, as effectively addressing cross-contact requires considering various perspectives, such as whether someone keeps their allergens in their home and where they fall on the food reactivity spectrum. Combining creative thinking, food allergy education, careful planning, and community advocacy can significantly reduce reactions and improve our safety regarding food allergies.

Awareness of cross-contact risks is vital, especially for individuals with anaphylactic allergies, as even the slightest trace of an allergen can trigger a life-threatening reaction. This underscores the importance of maintaining vigilance and meticulous attention to food preparation and handling, striving for safety without living in constant fear.

Key Strategies for Effective Allergy Management

Managing food allergies isn't about a single rulebook for everyone to follow; it's about building a toolkit you can rely on in daily life. The strategies below are designed to keep you safe, empowered, and adaptable, no matter what situations you encounter.

- Education and Advocacy: Education and advocacy play a significant role in creating a safer environment for yourself and others in the food allergy community. By educating those around you about cross-contact risks in ways that feel natural to you, you contribute to a broader understanding and safer practices.

- Emergency Preparedness: Despite our best efforts to prevent cross-contact, accidental exposure can still happen. Carrying necessary medications like antihistamines and epinephrine, knowing how to use them, and letting others you trust know how to use them will set you up for success in the event of a reaction. If you need help accessing epinephrine, please contact me via my website. I'm happy to assist with troubleshooting, help you research available options in your state, and connect you to an expert.

- Regular Review and Adaptation: Boundaries can and should evolve as you learn and grow. Regularly review and adapt your cross-contact prevention strategies as you encounter new environments, gain a deeper understanding, or if you encounter a change in your allergies. It's natural for accommodations to shift over time, and if others question these changes, you can explain that adapting boundaries is simply part of living with a food allergy.

Crafting a Personalized "Safe Products List"

If you have the time and energy, creating a "safe food product list" and a "safe non-food product list" can be highly valuable for sharing with friends, family, or anyone else who may need it. While labels can change, and your list might only sometimes be up-to-date, it can still guide people toward the brands you know and trust. Including typical stores where you buy these products in your list helps you and others use it effectively when shopping. For example, if a specific product is only available at one store in your city or online, having that information can save time and prevent unnecessary searching.

You can find examples of these lists on my website. They offer a quick way to share safe brands of foods and products I use when visiting someone's house, staying with them for a trip, or attending an event. These lists have been invaluable to me, and while creating them takes effort, it has been worth it for both myself and others.

While creating a safe product list isn't necessary for everyone, it can be a highly practical tool if you have the time. These lists offer significant value by managing food allergies more effectively, saving time, and providing clarity for you and those who support you or want to support you but aren't sure how.

Simple Strategies to Avoid Cross-Contact

While avoiding reactions due to cross-contact can be one of the trickiest parts of living with a food allergy, have no fear—there are practical steps you can take to make things easier and keep yourself safe. Here are my key strategies to help you avoid accidental exposure to allergens:

Cleaning Personal Items Regularly

Wiping frequently touched personal items like phones, keys, and reusable water bottles regularly with wet wipes or mild soap and water. I even take the extra step of washing or wiping the bottoms of my shoes now and then. It may seem silly, but avoiding tracking allergens into my home is worth it, especially if I've been in a super contaminated place!

Frequent Handwashing and Use of Wet Wipes

As previously mentioned, washing your hands with soap and water is the best way to protect against cross-contact. Wash for at least 20 seconds before and after eating to remove any food proteins. If you don't have access to soap and water, you can use wet wipes as a replacement. While wet wipes are helpful, they are less effective than sudsing up with soap and water.

Communicating Your Needs

It's essential to clearly explain the severity of your allergic reactions and the potential risks of cross-contact you watch out for so others can understand how to be cautious on your behalf. Sharing specific instructions on what to avoid and how they can assist in keeping you safe can look several ways, such as over text, a printed document for them to reference, etc. For example, I mentioned that my in-person workplace is kept free of my allergen, which is enforced by our HR department on my behalf in email blasts, flyers taped around the building in high-traffic areas, and verbal mentions from upper management every so often.

Requesting Accommodations in Public and Social Settings

As you can tell, accommodations for food allergies can vary widely. Emailing a restaurant or business ahead of time to ask about allergens works best for me, as it gives them a chance to focus on the details and ensures they have time to get back to me with accurate information. I will contact the host in advance for social gatherings to discuss the food and decide if I'm comfortable attending. If my allergen is involved in any capacity, I typically go only if I have a plan. I've had events and friends send out written reminders before get-togethers via text or email about keeping the space peanut-free, which I always appreciate.

Preparedness: Carrying Safe Snacks and Personal Utensils

I usually carry non-perishable, allergy-safe snacks around with me or to keep in my car just in case I end up in an unexpected situation—like finding myself at a restaurant I thought was safe but wasn't. If I'm eating at someone else's home, I may bring my own food, drink, utensils, dishware, and even a clean kitchen towel from my house. Depending on the circumstances, I may decide to wash their dishware and utensils myself with dish soap, using a fresh sponge to prevent cross-contact, and I often like to dry them with a disposable paper towel. I find that I will wash my hands frequently when in other spaces where my allergens are in use—it just depends on your preferences and what makes you feel comfortable and less anxious.

Having Emergency Medication Readily Available

Always carry at least two epinephrine medications, in case one is insufficient or has a misfire. I carry 4 since I've had to use more than two during anaphylaxis. With the exciting recent FDA approval of the first epinephrine nasal spray, epinephrine injections aren't the only option now, with additional advancements on the horizon as well that are needle-free.

Consider using temperature-controlled carrying cases designed for insulin and epinephrine to provide added protection since epinephrine degrades in certain temperatures. I use the brand Frio and have used my same insulated case for many years. It's also wise to keep antihistamines on hand for non-anaphylactic allergic reactions. Benadryl used to be the number one recommended antihistamine by allergists. However, Zyrtec and Allegra are often recommended by allergists instead due to fewer side effects.

Wearing a Medical ID Bracelet or Bag Tag

Medical ID jewelry is more than just an accessory—it can be a lifesaving precaution, especially when you're alone or around people who may not be familiar with your allergy. These bracelets can be customized with essential information to help you feel more secure. For example, mine clearly states my peanut allergy and that I always carry epinephrine in my purse.

In addition to wearable IDs, many smartphones now offer built-in medical ID features where you can store important health details like allergies, medications, and emergency contacts. There are also functional options like luggage tags, backpack and bag charms, and keychains that serve the same purpose of providing crucial information quickly, just in case it's ever needed because you can't speak for yourself.

Feeling Confident in Allergy Safety

By incorporating these strategies into your routine, you can better manage cross-contact risks and live with greater confidence. As we progress, it's worth considering how modern tools can further support your allergy journey. This brings me to my next section, where we'll explore various apps and technologies that help you navigate food allergies more effectively.

Tools and Technologies for Managing Food Allergies

After reflecting on my personal strategies for managing food allergies, I realized how technological innovation has added new layers of security. For many in the food allergy community, the development of specialized tools and digital solutions designed to enhance safety and convenience has significantly improved their lives.

Mobile apps like Fig and Allergy Force have emerged as valuable resources for individuals, offering features tailored to enhance safety and convenience. Fig, known for its comprehensive ingredient-checking capabilities, allows users to scan product barcodes and quickly assess allergen information. Similarly, Allergy Force not only assists in label scrutiny but also includes an emergency alert system—a feature that alerts designated contacts in case of a severe allergic reaction. While these apps provide robust support, the tool I use most often is Spokin.

Beyond locating allergy-friendly establishments, Spokin offers curated content ranging from travel tips to insightful interviews with food allergy influencers. This platform has become integral to my journey, offering practical guidance and a sense of community among allergy sufferers.

In addition, the internet has fostered numerous online communities dedicated to food allergies. These forums serve as invaluable resources for sharing experiences, accessing up-to-date information, and seeking support from others facing similar challenges. Whether discussing allergy management strategies or discovering new safe dining options, these communities offer a sense of solidarity and empowerment. Like any online group, there are pros and cons, but if you typically enjoy interacting with forums, online groups may be an option.

I have yet to fully embrace using apps for label checking or emergency alerts. As a millennial, I've already found my groove and had my methods down before most of the allergy apps came about. Still, I recognize their popularity among many in the allergy community. The evolution of these technologies continues to shape how individuals manage their allergies, promising even greater accessibility and functionality in the future, and I love that! I plan to investigate how I may use them more in the future.

Raising Awareness and Advocating for Change

Creating a safer environment for individuals with food allergies requires more than personal vigilance—it demands collective action and systemic change. Advocacy is crucial in promoting better practices in public spaces, from restaurants to schools and beyond. By encouraging proper training and education, we can work to reduce the risks associated with cross-contact and anaphylaxis, ultimately fostering a more inclusive and safer environment for everyone.

Promoting Allergy Practices in Public Places

Advocate for food allergy awareness in public spaces, including restaurants, schools, and other venues. Raising awareness in public spaces starts with understanding the real-world challenges individuals with food allergies face. Advocate for allergy-free zone signage if a business or place is purposefully allergen-free and transparent allergen information in places like restaurants, venues, and event spaces, both in person and on their website. Normalizing these practices can create environments where individuals with food allergies feel safer and more included.

Encouraging Allergy Awareness Training

Recommend proper training and food allergy education to reduce risks associated with cross-contact and anaphylaxis. Cross-contact and anaphylaxis pose serious risks, but effective food allergy education can mitigate these risks. Support mandatory training programs for employees in public places, emphasizing:

- Preventing cross-contact.
- Recognizing anaphylaxis signs.
- Administering epinephrine (both injectors and nasal sprays).

Training should address cleaning practices and emergency response procedures. Additionally, check your state's requirements for epinephrine on ambulances—many states do not mandate it—and ensure staff are well-informed to protect individuals with food allergies.

Advocating for standardized training is vital for creating safer environments. Support legislative efforts like the Restaurant Training Bill, Dillon's Law, Elijah's Law, the ADDE Act (SB 68), and the School Access to Emergency Epinephrine Act. Also consider backing Zacky's Bills—including Zacky's FAST Act, Zacky's Law, and the Muñoz SAFE Act—which were introduced through the efforts of a family that has staunchly championed stronger food allergy safety laws.

May is Food Allergy Awareness Month, with a designated Food Allergy Awareness Week during the month each year. These nationally recognized observances play a key role in raising public understanding, boosting visibility, and sending a message to elected officials that food allergy advocacy matters to their constituents. On my social media and website, I regularly share ideas for how to celebrate and how to request a proclamation recognizing Food Allergy Awareness Week in your state or city. It's easier than you might think! In fact, for almost any cause you care about—whether it's food allergies, LGBTQ+ rights, or environmental justice—you can often find proclamation templates online by searching "[your cause] + proclamation."

It's also worth noting that proclamations are typically issued on a yearly basis and do not automatically renew—so it's important to keep requesting them each year to maintain awareness and visibility.

Implementing Clear Allergen Labeling

Support initiatives that require clear and detailed labeling of allergens and PAL on packaged foods. Transparent and accurate allergen labeling is a non-negotiable for safety and advocating for legislation that mandates clear and comprehensive labeling on all packaged foods is paramount. This includes the presence of allergens and also the risk of cross-contact. By supporting these types of initiatives, we can help ensure that individuals with food allergies have the information they need to make safe food choices. Raising awareness about these gaps and advocating for stricter regulations can help prevent allergic reactions caused by misleading labels.

Acknowledging the Need for Unified, Community-Led Advocacy in the Allergy Space

The concept of having an allergy "threshold" is coming up more frequently, especially in conversations about Precautionary Allergen Labeling (PAL) and emerging policy decisions. As you've seen throughout this book, allergy testing and allergy management is far from perfect. From my limited but growing knowledge, having been part of ongoing PAL conversations in the allergy space, I'm hearing more and more talk about "thresholds" being used in future food labeling, often tied to something called the ED05.

An ED05 amount is referred to as an "eliciting dose," meaning it is the dose that triggers an objective allergic reaction. Exposure at or below the ED05 of allergenic foods has been shown to cause only mild to moderate symptoms in a small proportion of the allergic population. I personally don't believe this is the right approach. Discussions around ED05 often rely heavily on mathematical modeling to estimate allergen contamination risk, rather than on individual testing or on-site facility assessments. Additionally, these models don't account for the real-world scenario where someone will be consuming multiple products containing trace amounts of allergens, leading to cumulative exposure. This is especially concerning given how our bodies' responses can be influenced by co-factors, like hormones, stress, and sleep, which I discussed in Chapter 1, and these factors aren't typically considered in such assessments.

Many others I've spoken to in the food allergy community share my view that more extensive surveying of people with allergies is needed to develop a better, more effective action plan beyond ED05. The main reason is that this kind of labeling won't change how most of us attending these allergy conferences eat. In fact, it may cause confusion for those trying to learn their personal allergen threshold but finding it difficult or impossible to do so. We rely heavily on labels to be accurate and reliable for our safety, and this approach seems instead aimed at people who already aren't hyper-vigilant about labels—likely because their reactivity levels tend to be lower. This leaves out the needs of the most sensitive individuals and doesn't address the broader allergic population effectively. There are studies available on ScienceDirect and NIH's PubMed that explore ED01, ED05, ED10, and related topics for those interested in learning more.

What concerns me most is that these policies are being discussed in silos—coming from different directions, often without input from the very people who would be most affected. There are more than 33 million Americans with food allergies, and over 60 million with allergic conditions more broadly who may be reliant on these labels. The food allergy community, especially those living with these conditions day in and day out, reading and relying on labels, must be consulted in shaping food labeling policy. Anything less misses the mark.

What we need more than ever is unity, and most importantly, leadership that comes from those who live with allergies themselves. Policy change should be by the people, for the people—

not politically driven by entities seeking accolades, external validation, or something else. When those directly impacted lead the conversation, the policies reflect genuine needs and create meaningful, lasting impact.

Passing Policy to Ensure Allergy-Safe Measures

As an allergy community, we have to support legislation that enforces strong allergen management practices across the food industry, protecting millions of people affected by food allergies and other dietary restrictions, many of whom rely on accurate labeling and safe practices every day. I tend to get my information from social media allergy accounts and from trusted organizations like FAACT who provide updates on current bills, emerging research, and relevant statistics that keep the community informed.

I firmly believe it's essential to get involved locally and at the state level by working directly with representatives to champion food allergy legislation. Attend town halls, write to elected officials, and partner with advocacy groups to keep food allergy issues front and center on the legislative agenda.

Together, we can build a future where allergy safety is a priority, and advocacy is led by those who understand firsthand what's at stake. Support legislation that enforces strong allergen management practices across the entire food industry. Follow trusted organizations like FAACT to stay updated on current bills, emerging research, and relevant statistics that impact the food allergy community.

Get involved at the local and state level by working with representatives to champion food allergy legislation. With over 33 million Americans affected, food allergies are a serious public health issue and not just a niche concern. Engaging with policymakers is essential. Attend town halls, write letters or emails to your elected officials, and partner with advocacy groups to keep food allergy issues on the legislative agenda. The more of us who speak up, the louder our message becomes. That's how we move closer to meaningful change.

Participating in Community Food Allergy Education Initiatives

Leverage social media and local media outlets to share stories, tips, and information about managing food allergies. Social media is a powerful tool for raising awareness and educating the public. Use platforms like Instagram, TikTok, and Facebook to share your personal stories, offer tips, and spread information about food allergy management. Engaging with local media outlets can also amplify your message, reaching a wider audience and driving community action.

Educational content like videos, infographics, downloadable and printable pamphlets and posters can effectively spread awareness. Consider creating and sharing content that explains the importance of cross-contact prevention, proper allergen labeling, and emergency response. Collaborate with local schools, community centers, and online platforms to distribute these resources, helping to educate others and foster a more informed community.

By taking these practical steps and advocating for broader changes, we can foster a safer, more inclusive environment for individuals with food allergies. Whether through policy changes, public awareness campaigns, or community education, each action contributes to a more substantial movement toward inclusivity and safety for all.

Encouraging Businesses to Adopt Allergy-Friendly Measures

Creating safer environments for individuals with food allergies involves both public and private sector efforts. Businesses play a pivotal role in reducing allergen risks and enhancing safety. By implementing proactive measures and embracing best practices, they can significantly improve the quality of life for consumers with food allergies.

Establishing Allergy-Free Zones

Advocate for creating designated top allergy-free zones in public spaces, such as schools, libraries, gyms, event venues, daycares, and salons. These zones could include food-free areas and designated spaces where food can be consumed, reducing the risk of airborne allergens or cross-contact reactions.

While this concept is a personal dream inspired by my experiences with food allergies, I believe it is essential to create environments where individuals like me can feel secure and included. And recently, I've seen others in the space, like Mia Silverman, a popular allergy advocate, asking for it, too! Normalizing these areas could significantly enhance safety and comfort in public spaces for those affected by food allergies and it opens more discussion around accommodations and allergy education and awareness.

Designing Menus with Allergy Transparency in Mind

While comprehensive food labeling laws in the US have not yet kept pace with the needs of the food allergy community, there is powerful potential for progress. Advocates, leaders, and forward-thinking businesses are already pushing for change, and hopefully, the laws will continue to evolve to reflect these growing efforts. In the meantime, restaurants and bars can take meaningful steps by offering ingredient transparent menus and taking proactive measures to minimize cross-contact in their kitchens. Providing detailed allergen information and minimizing cross-contact in kitchens not only enhances safety, but it also builds trust and a loyal customer base. By drawing inspiration from places with stronger labeling practices, such as the EU, or legislation like California's Allergen Disclosure and Dining Experience (ADDE) Act, the US can take strides toward a more inclusive and informed dining culture.

I dream of a future where allergens are clearly marked on menus in a consistent way across the board, so that dining out becomes safer, easier, and more welcoming for all. Once those foundations of allergen transparency are in place, the US can take it a step further by disclosing full ingredient lists and being upfront about cross-contact risks.

If food manufacturers were required by policy to share more detailed cross-contact information, it would allow restaurants, bars, bakeries, and other food businesses to better assess and communicate risk—not from a liability standpoint, but from a place of informed decision-making. This would give customers with food allergies the ability to more accurately weigh their options and choose what feels safest for them.

Allergy Training in Food Service

Creating a safer dining experience for people with food allergies requires both clear menu labeling and proper staff training. Doing so sends an important message: that transparency matters, and that safety isn't optional. Everyone deserves allergen awareness to be a standard part of the dining experience. We all deserve to know what we're eating, and making allergen disclosure a requirement is a pivotal step toward ensuring that happens.

It's important to have legislation to make this a requirement and not optional, as restaurant policies in the US are governed at the state level, meaning there's no federal law from Congress overseeing this. Therefore, we have to push for change state by state, the same way we do for school legislation, which is state by state. In Kentucky, I've tried advocating for improvements, and I can tell you firsthand: it's hard to get our representatives of Congress on board since there are so many topics and areas of focus people want prioritized.

That's why statewide laws mandating restaurant staff training in allergen protocols and anaphylaxis response are so crucial. If there's no type of Restaurant Training Bill where you live, consider joining or starting advocacy efforts for one. These bills should cover essential practices like preventing cross-contact, recognizing the signs of anaphylaxis, knowing how to administer epinephrine (in all forms), and effectively responding during allergic reactions.

Several US states have enacted legislation requiring allergen awareness training in restaurants to help improve food allergy safety. Massachusetts led the way with its Food Allergy Awareness Act, mandating that restaurants post food allergy awareness information in staff areas, include menu notices urging customers to disclose allergies, and ensure that certified food protection managers complete allergen training.

Rhode Island followed with a nearly identical law. Illinois passed legislation requiring all food service establishments to have at least one certified manager trained in allergen awareness, while Michigan's Public Act 516 includes allergen safety in its required training for certified food safety managers. In Virginia, House Bill 2090 added food allergy training to the state's health department regulations for restaurants. Maryland requires restaurants to display a food allergy awareness poster for employees, and New York City mandates posters in multiple languages to reach a broader audience.

Even on the city level, places like Saint Paul, Minnesota, have adopted similar requirements. These efforts reflect growing recognition of the need for consistent allergen protocols in food service across the board in all states, not only to improve safety but to increase awareness and accountability. If you're unsure where to start, advocates can look to these examples as models when pushing for similar legislation in other states and talk to a food allergy organization about if initiatives are already in progress and to find out how to get things started. Together, allergen menu labeling and comprehensive staff training create a culture of safety and trust for those with food allergies while dining out.

Businesses and Influencers Can Raise Food Allergy Awareness

If you have a platform—big or small—you have the power to make a real difference in food allergy and anaphylaxis awareness. Encourage others to leverage their social media and business platforms for food allergy and anaphylaxis awareness. Businesses and individuals can amplify their impact by participating in education campaigns, sharing information about food allergies, and partnering with advocacy groups or influencers.

Collaborating with organizations and celebrities can help reach a broader audience and promote food allergy safety. Whether it's joining education campaigns to raise awareness, using social media to share tips and personal stories, working with advocacy groups to expand outreach, or engaging public figures to boost visibility, every effort counts. Promoting best practices such as improved allergen labeling, ongoing staff training, and emergency preparedness in public spaces can make a real difference.

By adopting these allergy-aware measures, businesses contribute to a safer and more inclusive environment. Creating designated allergy-friendly zones, offering clearer menu options, ensuring staff are trained continuously, and using your platform to raise awareness around the gravity of anaphylaxis all play vital roles in protecting individuals with food allergies and improving public safety.

Building Toward Comprehensive Allergen Legislation

I believe that the passage of improved food labeling laws will be the cornerstone for broader legislation, ultimately leading to cohesive and consistent restaurant menus that accurately reflect allergen content—and potential cross-contact risks.

Currently, businesses and consumers face significant challenges in accessing the information needed to make informed decisions about food safety. That's why improving food labeling laws from food manufacturers should be a top priority. Once these foundational laws are established, we can shift our focus to more specialized cross-contact training.

In the recent past—just nine months ago—I would've immediately recommended reaching out to FARE's advocacy department. I personally relied on them almost constantly for legal questions and policy guidance, and they were an invaluable resource for many in the food allergy community. However, with the recent shift in leadership and the sudden loss of their advocacy team, many of us who championed the organization have been left in the dark about whether advocacy is still a priority of theirs at all. It's disappointing not to have that reliable point of contact anymore, especially since so many of us had strong working relationships with their team.

That said, there are still fantastic organizations you can turn to for guidance. I recommend CFAAR, AAFA, ACAAI, AAAAI, and FAACT. I've learned a ton from FAACT's Roundtable Podcast, which covers all aspects of living with food allergies in their over 200+ episodes. Eleanor at FAACT started Camp TAG because she couldn't find a day camp that could guarantee safety for her own children, and she wanted siblings to attend together, whether allergic or not—Camp TAG would have been a dream for me as a kid growing up. On top of that, FAACT's website has an Inclusion Resource Center, full of free resources and exercises designed to help us all grow in more inclusive ways. If you're unsure where to start, I'm happy to help connect you—just reach out through my website, and I'll do my best to point you toward the right tools and people.

I truly hope FARE's leadership can regain the trust it once earned and restore its role as a non-profit the food allergy community can confidently rely on, as it did in the past. In the meantime, we keep moving forward together, supporting one another and continuing to push for safer, more inclusive practices. One of the most impactful areas we can improve is restaurant staff training on allergen protocols and ingredient transparency, which lays critical groundwork for safer dining experiences. For restaurants looking to implement stronger safety policies or explore established training programs, there are still organizations—hopefully FARE included—that can offer foundational guidance and up-to-date information.

Closing Thoughts & Additional Context

- Advocacy Organizations and Laws Advancing Food Allergy Safety: Several advocacy organizations and laws are making important strides to improve safety and awareness around food allergies:

    The Allison Rose Foundation was established in memory of Allison Rose Suhy, who tragically died from anaphylaxis caused by a peanut allergy. The foundation focuses on education, awareness, and prevention efforts, and actively supports policies such as the "Allison Rose Act" (House Bill 231). This legislation encourages schools to implement food allergy training programs for both staff and students. More information is available at allisonrosefoundation.org.

    Dillon's Law is named after Dillon Mueller, a young adult from Wisconsin who died from an anaphylactic reaction not to food, but after being stung by a bee. This law promotes legislation designed to enhance emergency response protocols and raise anaphylaxis awareness within schools and communities. It allows any individual in Wisconsin to be trained in the use of epinephrine, obtain it, and learn to use it to save a person's life. All people involved are covered from liability under the state's

Good Samaritan liability law. Other states have created versions of Dillon's law in their states.

The Elijah-Alavi Foundation and Elijah's Law work to increase food allergy education, improve access to emergency medications like epinephrine, and provide support for families affected by food allergies. Their initiatives aim to create safer environments in schools, businesses, and public spaces across the country.

- Cross-Contact is Not Small: The tragic June 2025 loss of recent Rhode Island college graduate Timmy Howard is a heartbreaking reminder that cross-contact is not minor and can be deadly. Just a week after celebrating his graduation, Patty and Tim Howard lost their son to anaphylaxis after he ate a candy bar that had peanut cross-contact. He had missed the "may contain" warning that was printed on the candy bar's label before buying it for a late-night snack, a mistake any of us can make, as we're all human. His family acted immediately, multiple epinephrine were administered, yet cross-contact still claimed his life. The focus is not which candy bar it was, but that it could have been any brand at any time because of our lack of labeling laws. Cross-contact is real and life-threatening for some, and Timmy's story underscores why fears around it are valid and why meaningful change is urgently needed.

- Heads-Up to Restaurants: It's important for restaurants to realize that turning away one person with allergies can mean losing their entire social network—family, friends, and colleagues—who might otherwise come along. Conversely, when a restaurant does well with allergy accommodations, it gets shared across the food allergy community network and their circles tend to flock to it the same way we do to a safe, trusted food brand. As a community, we are loyal customers!

- Getting Curious: Navigating the complexities of food allergies demands an ongoing commitment to awareness, particularly regarding cross-contact risks. Despite my 30+ years of experience, I continue to discover new and unexpected ways in which cross-contact can occur, highlighting the need for constant vigilance and proactive measures. By fostering a mindset of continuous learning, advocating for change, and remaining vigilant but not fearful, we can collectively create safer environments for individuals with food allergies, building a more aware and considerate community.

- Reading Labels: My approach to reading US food labels involves three key steps: checking the ingredients list, seeking facility-level allergen information, and consulting the brand's website or contacting the company if needed. Due to the lack of transparent facility-level labeling for allergens on shared equipment and in shared facilities, food shopping can be challenging for those with allergies, often requiring visits to multiple stores and extensive online research.

- Policy Wording: A major issue I've noticed in food allergy policy, and in policy across the board, is that laws are often passed as optional. When no one is required to implement them, nothing happens, and the effort to get them passed as mandatory has to start all over again. The same applies to language in policy—it's often written to be specific, which is necessary, but it also means if it is too specific, updates and new legislation are constantly needed, like with new epinephrine devices that aren't traditional injections. Now past policies in place are needing to be re-written and passed again to include non-injectable forms on the market. Something to consider when working on policy: make it mandatory, and think ahead to avoid language or requirements that could quickly become outdated.

- Dr. Rubin's Book: For anyone looking to expand their

knowledge on allergies and related conditions, a great resource is Dr. Zachary Rubin's upcoming book, *All About Allergies: Everything You Need to Know About Asthma, Food Allergies, Hay Fever, and More,* coming out in February 2026. Dr. Rubin is a board-certified allergist whose informative online content I love following, and his book covers a wide range of topics, all grounded in expert research.

- Call to Action: We must advocate for stricter food labeling laws in the US, including mandatory facility-level allergen information, enforceable consequences for non-compliance, and restrictions on misleading front-of-packaging claims. Implementing practices similar to those in the EU, Australia, South Korea, and Canada would assist in safeguarding the physical and mental health of individuals with food allergies and managing them. As it stands, inadequate labeling laws contribute to preventable allergic reactions, anxiety, and even fatalities—issues that could be mitigated with stronger legislation.

8

ACCOMMODATIONS

10 Practical Steps to Cultivate an Accommodation Mindset

Accommodations are essential for ensuring that individuals can participate fully and equally in all aspects of life. Recognizing that "disability" isn't a bad word but a reality that any of us could confront at any moment due to illness, injury, or simply aging, is vitally important. Disability rights are fundamental human rights, and advocating for accessible environments and inclusive practices is not just needed—it's a moral imperative that benefits everyone.

Healthcare is another fundamental human right, vital for supporting everyone, including those with disabilities. Ableism—discrimination against people with disabilities—is pervasive in society. I try to consciously reflect on and challenge my internalized ableism. We can move towards a more inclusive and compassionate world for all by confronting these biases.

Cultivating an accommodation mindset is essential for creating inclusive and supportive environments for everyone, including those with disabilities, food allergies, or other needs requiring specific accommodations. While these practices may take time to learn, the key is maintaining an open and proactive approach to support and include others.

Accommodations are sometimes stigmatized due to misunderstandings or a lack of awareness about the needs of those who require them. This stigma can appear as misconceptions, stereotypes, or a perceived burden on those providing accommodations. I find that embracing an accommodation mindset and promoting inclusivity is an ongoing process of learning and growth. Working together to reduce stigma can create environments where everyone feels valued. Here are 10 practical steps to help us all contribute to this goal:

1. Educate Yourself: Learn about various needs, such as food allergies, disabilities, and other conditions requiring accommodations. Understanding that everyone's accommodation preferences can differ is foundational for providing personalized support. Try to put yourself in someone else's shoes or do a quick Google search before asking questions that could quickly be answered. It can be exhausting for someone needing the accommodations to share the same resources and information repeatedly. Remember, people don't need to disclose private medical details in order for their accommodation to be taken seriously.

2. Listen Actively: Pay close attention to the needs and concerns of others. When someone is willing and comfortable to share and be vulnerable, validate their experiences by listening without judgment. Just as important, recognize that the people most impacted by an issue should be the ones guiding the solutions, and let their voices lead the change.

3. Communicate Clearly: Engage in open discussions with individuals about their needs and how you can best support them. Don't hesitate to ask for clarification if you're unsure, and always approach these conversations with empathy and a willingness to learn.

4. Plan and Prepare: Anticipate potential challenges and plan accordingly. This could involve researching safe dining options, identifying brands that offer allergen-free or accessible products, and ensuring spaces are accessible for everyone. Additionally, consider creating contingency plans for unexpected situations, such as bringing extra supplies or identifying alternative options to ensure everyone's needs are met. Being proactive in your

planning demonstrates your commitment to inclusivity and preparedness.

5. Create Inclusive Environments: Strive to make all spaces—whether at home, work, or social settings—safe and accessible for everyone. This might involve removing allergens, providing ramps, or ensuring clear signage. It's okay if you're unsure about the specific accommodations needed initially; reviewing your space and making some preliminary changes is a great start. A valuable second step is to ask those who visit regularly and have specific needs what would make them comfortable and safe in your space.

6. Stay Flexible: Be open to adjusting plans and routines to accommodate others. Flexibility is key when navigating life with a disability or other needs that might fall outside of societal norms. Demonstrating a genuine commitment to inclusivity and trying is more important than getting everything perfect from the start. Most of us won't get it right immediately, and that's okay.

7. Advocate for Inclusivity: Speak up for the needs of others in various environments like workplaces, schools, and public spaces. Advocate for policies and practices that guarantee everyone's safety and comfort. Stay informed about relevant bills and policies in your area that impact the rights of individuals with disabilities or other accommodation needs.

8. Educate Others: Share your insights about accommodations with friends, family, and colleagues. By raising awareness and providing information on various needs, you contribute to building a more understanding community.

9. Empower and Support: Encourage others to confidently voice their needs and advocate for themselves if they choose to. Provide support by being a reliable ally and resource.

10. Reflect and Improve: Regularly assess your approach to accommodating others. Seek feedback and be open to making improvements to better meet their needs. Remember that accommodations and individual needs can evolve, so ongoing reflection and checking in is integral.

Effectively addressing accommodation requests involves understanding legal obligations, engaging in interactive dialogue and active listening, and implementing reasonable solutions. Ultimately, creating an inclusive environment benefits everyone. Next, we will explore strategies for handling accommodation refusals and navigating potential conflicts.

10 Practical Steps to Mitigate Lack of Accommodation

Despite our best efforts to cultivate inclusive and supportive environments, there will inevitably be instances where accommodation requests are met with refusal. This reality can be incredibly challenging for individuals with food allergies, disabilities, or other specific needs. Not only does a refusal impact the practical aspects of accommodating someone, but it can also take a significant mental toll, leaving individuals feeling undervalued, overlooked, and isolated. Here are some practical steps to address and manage these challenges when they arise:

1. Educate Yourself and Others: Gain a thorough understanding of the legal rights and regulations related to accommodations. Familiarize yourself with the specific laws and guidelines that apply in various settings, such as workplaces, schools, or public venues. Share this knowledge to raise awareness about the responsibilities and importance of providing accommodations. Note that regulations vary by context, and some areas may not have specific rules, leading to more frequent accommodation refusals. For example, airlines do not adhere to the same ADA

(Americans with Disabilities Act) requirements as other sectors in the US, which impacts their handling of accommodations. This explains why airlines might disregard ADA requirements when refusing to accommodate food allergies or mishandling mobility aids like wheelchairs without repercussions.

2. Communicate Clearly: If you need accommodations, clearly articulating your specific needs and explaining why they are essential can be very helpful. Using clear, concise language and providing relevant examples to illustrate how the accommodations impact your well-being or ability to participate fully can make a significant difference. While it's unfortunate that the responsibility often falls on the person needing accommodations, taking the time to provide context can help others better understand and support your needs. By striving to express your needs clearly, you increase the likelihood of receiving a positive response in situations where you must advocate for yourself.

3. Document Requests: Keep detailed written records of all accommodation requests and responses. I try to get things in writing as much as possible, such as an email with a date and time, so I have a clear trail to reference if needed. This documentation can be crucial for addressing any surprise refusals and helping advocate for necessary changes.

4. Seek Support: Connect with relevant advocacy groups, legal advisors, or support networks for guidance and assistance in securing your accommodations. It's also perfectly okay to seek support from therapists or other professionals who can provide emotional and practical help. Having a support system in place can make a significant difference in navigating these challenges.

5. Propose Solutions: When faced with resistance, try to offer practical and feasible solutions while maintaining a calm

demeanor. I know first-hand how challenging and energy-draining it can be to request accommodations and explain their reasoning, especially over time. However, being open to possible solutions can facilitate negotiation, compromise, and find a middle ground. Sometimes, this approach uncovers accommodations I had yet to consider, but they have proven effective, and I can now ask for them again and again moving forward. *Silver linings.*

6. Follow-Up: If initial requests are denied, follow up with additional information or alternative solutions. Persistence is often key to overcoming refusals. Ask to speak to another point of contact. For example, I've found it helpful to email with a message like, "Do you have someone in your life with a food allergy? If not, could you direct me to someone else who might understand this better? Thank you." While this approach doesn't guarantee that the next person will fully grasp your experience, it's worth trying. Another option is to request a conversation with a manager or another decision-maker who may be able to assist further.

7. Escalate When Necessary: If your reasonable requests are continuously denied, you can escalate the issue to higher authorities or regulatory bodies. Ensure you follow the appropriate channels and procedures, which will vary depending on the situation.

8. Raise Awareness: Educate the broader community about the importance of accommodating others and the potential consequences of refusal. These consequences include increased physical and emotional stress, reduced participation, legal issues, strained relationships, lowered morale, missed business opportunities, reputational damage, exclusion, worsened health outcomes, and financial costs. Raising awareness can foster greater support and compliance in the future.

9. Leverage Technology: Use assistive technologies or other tools to bridge gaps when accommodations are not immediately available. These can offer temporary solutions and demonstrate the feasibility of permanent accommodations. For example, I will wear an N95 or KN95 mask to help manage my peanut allergy when accommodations are not provided, such as on public transit or in shared spaces like doctor's offices or hospitals. Additionally, recording and sharing your experiences—whether of inadequate or exceptional accommodations—on social media or with relevant parties can highlight the issues or successes in accommodation practices. This approach can help raise awareness and promote improvements.

10. Reflect and Adjust: Continuously evaluate the effectiveness of your approach to accommodations. Be open to feedback and willing to adapt your strategies to better address and mitigate refusals; I've learned a great deal from doing so. Asking trusted friends who don't have the same accommodations for their perspectives can provide valuable insights. This approach often leads to better solutions and demonstrates mutual support and understanding.

Navigating accommodation refusals calls for a proactive and multi-faceted game plan. Think of it as a toolkit: educate yourself and others, aim to keep communication as straightforward as possible, document when it feels important to you, and don't hesitate to seek support. As I transition into sharing my personal accommodation stories, remember that persistence and adaptability are your best friends when tackling accommodation challenges and prioritizing your own self-compassion and self-care.

My Personal Journey

I won't sugarcoat it—writing this section was overwhelming. Recounting experiences where accommodations were refused or mishandled stirred emotions I wasn't expecting. Reflecting on these instances, I recognize that my communication could have been clearer in some situations. However, it's important to note that not all of my accommodation challenges were within my control—not by a long shot. I was met with outright rudeness by many of them who were responsible for accommodating me.

Similar to my reflections on experiencing anaphylaxis in Chapter 4, I share these personal stories to reassure others that they are not alone in their accommodation requests, successes, and struggles. This section focuses on the workplace—a familiar setting for many of us—where I manage my life-threatening, airborne food allergy among 40+ employees and a few well-behaved office pups who brighten my days (from a distance to avoid any contamination).

When comparing my first workplace accommodation for my peanut allergy in 2008 to today, I see immense improvement, which fills me with hope and a warm-fuzzy feeling of being a valued employee and part of a community. This progress stems from a combination of better communication and increased confidence in articulating my needs. Still, I believe the primary difference is due to society's growing awareness of food allergies. Nowadays, when I disclose my food allergy as a disability during job interviews and advocate for a peanut-free environment, I'm usually pleasantly surprised by how smooth these discussions go.

In contrast, when I was growing up, my time in school pre-dated Section 504 plans for food allergies, and skepticism about the severity of my allergy was prevalent—even within the medical community. There simply wasn't as much data or awareness around food allergies and anaphylaxis collected as there is today. I used to worry that disclosing my food allergy might hinder my chances of being hired, but time and again, I've found the opposite to be true. People appreciate my transparency, and I take pride in presenting myself authentically during interviews and advocating for my needs. If a potential employer can't accommodate me, I'd rather know their stance upfront.

I wholeheartedly support peanut-free and nut-free schools. What a dream it would've been to have that as an option growing up. I often wonder how much that kind of environment would've changed my confidence, my relationships, and even my sense of safety on a daily basis. Spending over a decade of your life in a place you have to be—five days a week, nine months a year—shouldn't come with the constant threat of a life-threatening reaction. The peace of mind that nut-free policies could provide to nut-allergic students, families, and even teachers is something I deeply value. I once thought I couldn't become a teacher because of my peanut allergy and ruled it out as a child, assuming it would never be a safe career path for me. Now, I think I could actually work at one of these schools.

I've heard figures in the allergy community argue against nut-free environments, saying it unfairly singles out certain allergens or that avoiding exposure doesn't teach children necessary life skills. I understand that perspective, but I also think it overlooks the day-to-day reality of food allergy management and the mental load involved. For a child with anaphylactic nut allergies, being able to learn without that constant fear in the background can be life-changing. One in 13 children has a food allergy today, and one in 10 adults—meaning roughly 10% of students entering college are managing this. It's not rare, and I love that nut-free schools are now an option that can serve as a legitimate and life-affirming accommodation for some families.

Peanut-free, nut-free, and hybrid schools can help raise allergy awareness for students with allergies, which is another reason I support them, but they are *not the only solution* for accommodating allergens—not at all! For those with milk, egg, wheat, and other allergens, accommodations need to be provided as well. Nut allergies aren't inherently more "severe," "important," or "common" than other allergens, so all allergens deserve equal consideration and support. If there are multiple allergens, classrooms can be adjusted accordingly to meet the needs of each individual.

Practices put in place for peanut or tree nut allergies, like hand-washing after eating in the cafeteria to remove allergens and prevent the spread of germs, can also be leveraged to support other food allergies, helping ensure they are taken seriously too. A peanut-free school would allow me to work in a school setting, but accommodations shouldn't stop there—finding how all the different supports come together is key. I do support these accommodations, but let me be clear: "nut-free" and "peanut-free" does not automatically mean "allergy-friendly."

As an adult with food allergies, I've reflected on this quite a bit since it is a hot topic in the allergy space, and I've seen many people on social media oppose nut-free schools, even though as far as I have personally seen those individuals are not people with life-threatening cross-contact or airborne allergies themselves, and this is why I feel it is important to explain why calling out accommodations like no nuts in schools or no nuts on planes matters.

This is purely my opinion and not based on formal research, though studies in the EU on restaurant menus requiring allergen transparency have shown that such measures promote broader allergy awareness. We can't always please everyone, but prioritizing accommodations and allergy-aware spaces, like nut-free schools and gluten-free certifications for restaurants, benefits the community as a whole and helps those who rely on these spaces and programs to stay safe.

I'm in favor of calling out specific allergen-free spaces as they're needed, such as in schools, camps, restaurants, and workplaces. Being granular about needed accommodations is important. Since we cannot accommodate everyone all the time, we can still provide measures that protect people when needed, and having clear, realistic guidelines ensures that those who truly need protection are not overlooked.

Advocacy and policy change are part of what makes these environments possible. Tracking federal and state-level bills that support food allergy accommodations is one way to help ensure these options continue to expand. Supporting legislation and letting the voices of those most impacted guide these changes—and broader allergy accommodations—truly effective and transformative for everyone involved.

My first job after high school was in a large corporate building with hundreds of employees. I only disclosed my food allergy after receiving the job offer, and unfortunately, they barely made any accommodations. I asked that the break room and my section of the building be kept peanut-free, but my request was denied. Instead, I was told to ask each person around me not to eat peanuts, which was awkward, but something I attempted while being met with copious strange looks. I was also advised to eat lunch at my desk or in my car.

Despite my efforts to avoid the break room, I still experienced allergic reactions from cross-contact and once accidentally touched a sticky, peanut butter-like substance on the refrigerator door. After that, I stopped using the break room altogether and would only bring room-temperature meals to work that I could keep at my desk until lunchtime without it needing to be heated. It was far from ideal. That job offered the least accommodation I've ever experienced. Luckily, I've seen substantial improvement since then, with each subsequent job position providing significantly better support.

At a previous in-person job, my employer went above and beyond by swapping out the vending machine items to exclude peanuts—an accommodation request I hadn't even considered but absolutely loved. This experience reinforced the value of open conversations about accommodations. Just because I need them doesn't mean I always know the best solutions. I initially thought it would be too difficult to change out the vending machine items, but the vending machine company assured me it was a simple adjustment and no problem at all. However, it was denied when I made a similar request at my gym.

One of the more challenging aspects I face regarding workplace accommodations has been navigating career opportunities limited by my food allergy—for example, I wouldn't try to be a flight attendant even though it sounds fun. And, not that I want to, but I can't work at most food establishments. Obvious places like Texas Roadhouse or Five Guys are out of the question. Since I avoid environments where my allergen is prevalent or mostly unable to be controlled, it has restricted my options.

At my current job, travel opportunities with colleagues may arise, but I know I'd either need to decline or experience the trip differently, since it isn't one I'm planning myself. Meeting with clients and vendors would be required, and all the work of figuring out where I could safely go would fall on me. It would take a lot of time and energy, because I'm the only one who truly knows my allergy. These are times when my food allergy can feel like a weight on me just because I can't always be included or participate fully.

Also, peanut-containing products are strictly prohibited on-site. My employer tries hard to ensure my safety, providing a separate treat for celebrations and consulting me on suitable brands and restaurants. During team lunches or events, they ensure no peanuts are present in meals and arrange an alternative, safe meal for me. If necessary, I bring my own food, but their efforts make me feel valued. Though it's not flawless, their commitment and responsiveness when mistakes happen reaffirm their respect for my needs and the needs of others.

Here's an example showcasing my current employer's proactive approach. When scheduling an in-person interview after my initial remote one, they asked what measures they could take to ensure my safety. This thoughtful consideration immediately signaled that they valued my well-being and were willing to accommodate my needs. It was a reassuring moment that indicated the potential for a good fit between their company culture and my requirements.

These accommodations are like those at my previous employment, but my current company is much smaller. While my former employer occupied two floors of a building with 500 employees, my current workplace houses around 40 people in a more compact space. In smaller environments, in general, it's easier for everyone to adhere to a peanut-free or allergy-friendly policy. In the past, I had far more challenges with people bringing peanuts into the building and inadvertently contaminating common areas like door handles and elevator buttons by purposefully eating my allergen outside and then returning. Thankfully, this hasn't been an issue lately.

I always strive to be understanding when someone asks questions about my allergy, no matter how basic they seem—like whether peanut butter contains peanuts (a question I've gotten more than once). Instead of laughing, I see these inquiries as efforts to ensure my safety, especially in contrast to experiences where others have been indifferent or even deliberately disregarded my allergy. I also recognize that I may ask fundamental questions about others' needs when unfamiliar with their requests!

I previously served as the front desk associate at an art museum/hotel, and peanuts were used in the building, but not in my immediate workspace. Although it was a public-facing environment where patrons could bring in anything, causing occasional anxiety, I managed by stepping away when necessary and just letting others know why. However, I much prefer the controlled environment of my current workplace, where outside risks are greatly minimized.

When I worked as a floral designer, I loved the day-to-day tasks in the main florist building, but eventually I had to request a move to a smaller satellite location to maintain a peanut-free workspace. Despite this, I still faced challenges, like when the "floral processor" at the main branch would snack on peanuts while handling flowers, leading to inadvertent cross-contact issues. Fortunately, after discussing the matter, the issue was resolved easily, and he was very apologetic.

Allergen exposure can arise unexpectedly, so minimizing these risks has been crucial for me. Some might wonder, "Why does the entire building need to be free of the allergen?" But when I'm spending 8+ hours a day, 5 days a week in a space, having frequent allergic reactions that could be prevented just doesn't make sense.

I also recognize that I only manage one anaphylactic allergen, while others I know juggle 30+ allergies—some anaphylactic, some not—so an allergen-free space isn't a one-size-fits-all solution. I've faced similar questions about accommodations, like when flying: "Why does the whole plane need to be free of one person's allergen?" The reality is that living with a food allergy is exhausting, and the general public only sees a small slice of our constant need for accommodations. News flash: It's not just at work or on the plane—we're asking for these accommodations everywhere. I had to plan my own peanut-free wedding, for goodness' sake!

Hearing comments like, "Having a food allergy is your problem, not mine," or "They should get their own plane," or "No nuts on the entire plane just for one person? That's ridiculous!" makes my stomach turn. Sad to say, these attitudes are something I encounter far too often—both in person and online.

Even my hobbies have been affected by my allergy. For example, when renting an art studio in an open floor plan building, I faced significant issues with airborne allergens and cross-contact with others eating in nearby studios. I now practice glass torchwork and ask others in a studio to avoid eating peanuts while I'm there. Despite this accommodation, I often worry about cross-contact, especially since I know that they previously have eaten many peanut-containing snacks and peanut candies. It's similar at the local ceramics studio where I take classes and even at my gym. I can request accommodations, but that doesn't guarantee the space will be peanut-free or that the requests will always be followed.

While I haven't pushed the boundaries as much in my career and hobbies, I admire those who do and find that seeing their life experiences on social media really boosts my food allergy confidence.

In high school, I regularly volunteered in person at the Kentucky Humane Society, but I had to stop after experiencing repeated allergic reactions that resulted in hives. This was before I knew about cross-contact and how often peanut products are found in dog treats and toys.

While I still volunteer with them, it's now often in less direct ways. I used to love walking their senior dogs, and they've since added fun programs, like taking a dog out for a "date day," that I would love to be more involved with. These days, I primarily contribute by donating hand-painted pet portraits for their fundraisers and auctions, and I occasionally participate in events where they kindly set up a peanut-free zone for me to do things like face painting at their annual celebrations. They've candidly told me that they use peanut butter twice a day with the dogs, mostly because it's one of the most common donations they receive, not because it's essential. I'm grateful they consider peanut allergies even in small ways and were transparent with me about the actual risk and why switching to nut-free would be tricky as a not-for-profit.

Instead of assuming I can't be involved anymore, I've found creative ways to continue supporting the causes I care about, such as volunteering remotely or with accommodations that make it possible for me to show up safely.

I've found that firmly establishing boundaries, advocating for my needs, and staying adaptable in finding solutions have contributed significantly to my confidence and well-being, especially when navigating a world where my allergens are often present. No means no, and staying strong in my boundaries and not allowing them to be swayed takes practice when people are asking, "Can you just have a little bit?" The reality is no, I can't, and it is *not* worth it. By minimizing risks and managing my food allergies more effectively, I've experienced a happier and more fulfilling life. I've also found ways to give back, which is a core value of mine.

Missing Out & Having a Food Allergy Disability

Coming up in Chapter 11, I unpack the layered—and often overlooked—overlap between food allergies and mental health. Sadness and isolation often come with being unable to be accommodated in certain situations. It's okay to acknowledge that and to grieve it. My therapist has shared journaling prompts that help me navigate these tricky moments, especially when I feel overwhelmed or clouded by emotion.

Thankfully, I've found that stream-of-consciousness journaling brings clarity. It helps me untangle what I'm feeling and turn toward myself with self-compassion. It's a tool I reach for whenever I have to sit out because of my food allergy disability, but also beyond that—when I'm struggling with something else in life, feeling angry and unsure why, or simply needing to sit with an emotion and work through it.

I recently felt a range of emotions when a family member surprised us by saying they wanted to take us on a family vacation to Morocco. Initially, I felt elated and grateful, and I began looking into the culture there and what the trip might entail. Riding a camel through the Sahara Desert, exploring vibrantly tiled city streets, and seeing the towering mountain ranges of North Africa…I mean, *wow*. I got on my phone and searched for the travel website they planned to use. It was an all-inclusive company they had heard glowing reviews about and were generously offering to treat us to.

I scanned the itinerary. I opened the FAQs.

I scrolled through photos of the provided food.

And just like that… I knew I couldn't join. There was no way. Not safely. Not without an exhausting amount of planning, explaining, coordinating, and contingency-prepping. Not without draining every ounce of my energy just to try to make it work. The light in my mind that had lit up with possibility flickered, and then shut off.

As my eyes blurred with tears and traced the fine print of the tour package, a heavy ache settled in my chest. The words swam before me, but the message was clear. My tears came without my permission as I read: "10 nights in handpicked hotels, 10 breakfasts, 3 lunches, 6 dinners, 1 cooking class, 3 tastings, 14 sightseeing tours, private motor coach…" I just knew this wouldn't work for me. The level of accommodations required with a group of up to 22 travelers, being unable to pick my own meals or escape from the food they were providing, and managing cross-contact on a bus felt impossible. I couldn't feasibly see how to make it work and still be included.

It would have been an incredible opportunity to better connect with that side of the family, including my little niece, whom I adore and would have loved to travel alongside. The energy required by my husband and I to try to get these accommodations, knowing they might be denied and hard to get translated clearly into another language, just made me crumble. Not to mention, around this same time, a food allergy death happened in Morocco by someone who spoke the language fluently. Not to say it can't be done safely, but I was emotionally shaken up as all these thoughts flooded my mind while I sat in the restaurant trying to keep my cool. These are the emotional highs and lows you may hear about in the allergy community.

Whether I found a way to go, whether my husband and I booked a separate trip on our own, or something else, it's times like these when I feel envious about my allergy holding me back from experiences. Sometimes, I wonder if my needs are asking too much. I wish I could blend in without special accommodations, but that's not my reality. That's why I consider my cross-contact, airborne food allergy to be a disability. It is one for me, in the same way that others with varying disabilities navigate these spaces and daily challenges.

I share this to highlight the internal, invisible challenges that come with living with a food allergy. It's okay that I can't go, and I know I'm not alone—there are so many others in the disability community who require accommodations and have to miss out on things. But even knowing that, the sadness doesn't just disappear. Sometimes I need to let that sadness sit with me for a while as I work through it, honoring the feelings that come with missing out and the quiet losses that no one else sees.

I never thought of myself as "disabled" until I read American activist Judy Heumann's book *Being Heumann*, and I felt an internal click into focus, like a camera adjusting its lens just so. I couldn't put the book down, I was completely consumed by it. I re-read it soon after finishing because it resonated so deeply. I wanted to feel that feeling again—that sense of being understood, and of understanding parts of her. *Being Heumann* helped me realize that I had a disability, too, and it inspired me to start sharing this with people I knew so they could better understand me, and we could connect more deeply.

I highly recommend her book to everyone, disabled or not. Sadly, she passed away in 2023, but her global impact speaks volumes and will continue creating positive change forever. Her backstory is that in the early 1950s, she contracted polio as a child and became a wheelchair user. Because of this, she was later denied a teaching license in New York because she used a wheelchair. Officials told her that her disability would make her a "fire hazard" and that she wouldn't be able to evacuate students safely in an emergency. This injustice sparked her life-long fight for equality.

I discovered her story while watching a CBS Sunday Morning segment for the award-winning documentary called *Crip Camp*. The documentary, which includes footage from the 1970s and interviews with disability activists, highlights their pivotal role in advancing disability rights in the United States. I was shocked to learn how recent these changes were! The Americans with Disabilities Act (ADA) was passed the same year I was born, in 1990. The ADA Amendments Act followed in 2008, the same year I graduated high school. I was alive during disability history without even realizing it.

This 2008 amendment was crucial in getting food allergies recognized as a valid disability. It clarified that a condition doesn't always need to be actively symptomatic to qualify, which helped ensure that food allergies, despite being episodic, could still be covered under the ADA.

The ADA is the primary civil rights law that prohibits discrimination against people with disabilities in many aspects of public life. The disability rights movement continues today, advocating for equal rights. For instance, did you know that if you receive disability payments from the government, you can only have $2,000 in assets in total? I follow a woman on social media who shares her struggles with this issue, as her wheelchair-accessible van alone costs much more than that. This limitation is deeply offensive to those with disabilities, and thankfully, many activists are working to change it.

What I loved about both the film *Crip Camp* and Judy Heumann's book is the consistent tone of championing throughout, which underscores the relentless advocacy and leadership in the disability rights movement. Her vision was for the ADA to continue to keep up with societal changes, such as the internet and websites being accessible for people who are blind or low vision, as well as people who are deaf. She felt that, as a society, we need to have obligations to include everyone, and I think that same way, too. Inclusion for everyone is vital, as it ensures that all individuals, regardless of their abilities, have equal access to opportunities and resources, fostering a more just and equitable community.

For individuals with disabilities, such as food allergy disabilities or others, inclusion means being able to participate fully in social, educational, and economic activities, which enhances their quality of life. Inclusion not only benefits individuals with disabilities but also enriches society by embracing a wide range of perspectives and talents.

Additionally, inclusion helps break down stereotypes and prejudices, fostering greater empathy and understanding across the board. It encourages the development of more accessible and universally designed environments, which can benefit everyone. By promoting inclusion, society upholds human rights and dignity, ensuring people with disabilities are respected and valued as equal community members.

For anyone whose food allergy limits events, work, or travel, *Crip Camp* and *Being Heumann* may be deeply healing. These works underscore the importance of advocating for your needs and the profound impact of finding a supportive community. Judy Heumann's experiences and the activism depicted in *Crip Camp* demonstrate that fighting for accessibility and accommodations is necessary in achieving equality and inclusion for all disabilities, including those related to food allergies.

Between watching *Crip Camp* and reading Judy Heumann's memoir, I was cracked open to the transformative power of community. Together, they fit seamlessly in my understanding—like two pieces of a puzzle into place, revealing a fuller, clearer picture of the disability rights movement.

The film's powerful footage brought to life the activism that happened not so long ago, while Judy's story, told with raw honesty in both the film and her book, gave me a deeply personal window into overcoming discrimination and fighting for equality. These works are both educational and profoundly motivating, showing how collective action can spark real change. I can't recommend them enough.

To examine your own internalized ableism—something we all have, even those with disabilities—start by reflecting on your beliefs about disability and how societal norms have shaped them. Educate yourself on the history and experiences of disabled people, listen to their stories, challenge stereotypes, advocate for accessibility, and practice empathy to better understand their perspectives.

Learning about the history of disability rights in the US and realizing the movement is still very much ongoing inspired me to support the food allergy community in their policy efforts. That journey led me to discover the non-profit FARE (Food Allergy Research & Education) and get involved with their phenomenal advocacy team. Their guidance felt like hand-holding into advocacy—something I never thought I could do on my own until they showed me the way and gave me hope.

That's why I'm so distraught to see the organization seemingly shifting as of late, with leadership changes and the advocacy team no longer active on their website—without any clear explanation to the community. While their "Courage at Congress" event wasn't held in 2025, I used to look forward to it every year. It was an extraordinary initiative focused on legislative advocacy, with a team dedicated to educating and empowering the food allergy community, while demystifying the complex US legislative process.

Thankfully, other allergy organizations have developed similar Capitol Hill advocacy days. For example, Allergy & Asthma

Network has partnered with the American College of Allergy, Asthma and Immunology (ACAAI) to host an annual event known as "Allergy & Asthma Day on Capitol Hill." The Asthma and Allergy Foundation of America (AAFA) also does this type of federal outreach. On World Asthma Day in 2025, AAFA organizers and patient advocates visited Congressional offices in Washington, D.C., to highlight the needs of the more than 100 million people in this country who live with asthma or allergies. They also held a public awareness gathering outside the Capitol, in partnership with the American Academy of Allergy, Asthma, and Immunology (AAAAI), to help amplify the message and encourage policy support.

Advocating for bills protecting the food allergy community makes me believe in the possibility of a brighter future. I shouldn't have to consider moving abroad—such as to Europe, where food allergy legislation is more advanced—just to eat safely, leaving behind family, friends, and the life I know. Yet, many make this huge leap of moving across the globe for the fact that there is more transparency around allergens in other countries.

At a different food allergy conference last year, I asked a question during a session where a speaker was enthusiastically discussing advancements in allergy treatments and management. I share in that excitement—truly, progress in the field gives me hope. But I also felt the need to ask about the glaring inequities in our current system.

I made it clear that I'm only excited about advancements if they are accessible to everyone, not just those who can afford them. The speaker acknowledged the issue, but as a practitioner, admitted they had limited power beyond the scope of their individual work. In a striking moment that underscored the urgency of this problem, another audience member—a practicing physician—built on my point by sharing that he personally knows families who split the cost of a single two-pack of epinephrine, with one injector going to each allergic child or friend. This is the harsh reality: many people are going without epinephrine altogether due to cost, or are carrying only one injector, even though medical guidelines stress the importance of always having two in case of misfire or if the first dose isn't sufficient in managing the reaction.

This isn't just a policy issue—it's a life-or-death disparity. In our country where universal healthcare still isn't guaranteed, as it deserves to be as a basic human right, we must continue advocating for meaningful, structural changes that prioritize access and equity.

Our excitement for innovation must be grounded in a commitment to *inclusion.* "Be the change you wish to see," isn't just a feel-good quote—it's a call to action. If you're already taking steps toward that change, kudos to you. But if we truly want universal healthcare, we need to raise our voices and demand it. Too many people in the United States are still going without care, denied coverage, and, tragically, some are dying because of it.

Closing Thoughts & Additional Context

- Cultivating an Accommodation Mindset: Disability rights are fundamental human rights, and creating accessible environments benefits us all; whether now or in the future. Anyone can experience disability at any point in life, so understanding that accommodations are not special favors but essential tools for full participation and equality helps build a more inclusive, compassionate society.

- Education and Empathy: Take time to learn about the diverse needs of people with disabilities and marginalized communities and genuinely listen to their experiences and concerns. Approaching conversations with empathy and clear communication fosters understanding, builds trust, and ensures accommodations truly meet individual needs. I practice keeping an open mind and choosing to believe people when they share their truths and challenges.

- Creating Inclusive Environments: Efforts to create a safe and accessible space can make a tremendous difference. Since everyone's accommodation needs are unique, we can't assume or automatically know what will work best, and that's perfectly okay! Recognizing that we might not get it right the first time is part of the process, but the important thing is not to give up when things don't go perfectly. The real key is to ask openly and listen carefully. Clear communication about needs and preferences is essential, and staying flexible and willing to adjust plans demonstrates a genuine commitment to inclusivity and respect.

- Struggles with Accommodations: I know firsthand how stressful it can be when accommodations fall through or are refused. When that happens, it's natural to feel overwhelmed and frustrated, especially if other stressors are already weighing on you. But you're not alone in this. Many people face similar challenges, and persistence and advocacy can lead to real, positive change. By standing firm and seeking the accommodations you deserve, you not only support yourself but also help build a more accessible and inclusive world. Keep pushing forward when you can and remember that your voice and efforts matter because you're a part of a larger web, all connected and working together to create a more equitable environment for everyone.

- Workplace Accommodations: My journey from minimal accommodations in my first job to comprehensive support in my current role reflects not only progress in workplace inclusivity but also my growing confidence in advocating for myself. While I chose to be upfront about my food allergy during interviews and it led to positive outcomes with employers appreciating the transparency, it is important to remember that not everyone needs to disclose right away. What worked for me was following my instincts on what to ask for, so it is important to do what feels right for you. For me, this approach has helped create multiple workplace environments where I feel supported and where employers feel confident in ensuring my safety.

- Unlearning Ableism and Bias: You might be thinking, "I don't have any bias or internalized ableism." But I challenge that! Just like I've had to recognize that I live in a racist society—and that means I've internalized racism, too—I've also had to admit that I've internalized ableism. To continue to build on this, it's the same way I've had to challenge my own thoughts around consumption living in a capitalist society and trying to be more anti-capitalist, do less comparison, and really assess better what I need to be buying versus what I don't. None of this makes us bad people; it makes us human. We are all shaped by the biased systems in which we grow up, including racist, capitalist, and ableist ones. Reflecting on our personal beliefs about these topics and the influence of societal norms can help us begin to untangle those ideas we may believe are our own but are actually just something we internalized from around us. I've learned that internalized ableism often shows up as shame, self-doubt, or hesitation to ask for accommodations, and it affects both disabled and non-disabled people. When we examine these ingrained messages, we take powerful steps toward self-acceptance, stronger advocacy, and deeper inclusion—for ourselves and others.

I'll share a long quote, but one that's powerful and worth reading through. The Stimpunks Foundation's 2024 glossary defines *internalized ableism* as:

...prevalent in the wider world, but something that we often don't consider is the ableist views we hold about ourselves. It is inevitable that after spending our lives surrounded by normative culture, we become conditioned to view ourselves as broken, deficient, or less than. Despite being able to share compassion with others, we still harbour

overtly bigoted views towards ourselves. We internalise the harmful things said to us by our peers and professionals —sometimes even partners and friends. We take them all in and think less of ourselves and we begin to believe that there is something wrong with us.

Internalised ableism doesn't mean you are a bad person. It simply means you have turned negative messages about autism/disability in on yourself. This is not a conscious choice, it is a result of repeatedly experiencing or witnessing mistreatment and oppression of yourself and others over time. It doesn't mean you are ableist towards others or lack compassion for others.

- Disability Awareness: Recognizing that food allergies can be valid disabilities can provide a framework for understanding and advocating for necessary accommodations. Framing food allergies within the context of disability helps identify needed adjustments and advocate for equitable treatment and inclusive practices. To learn more, one place I suggest looking is Disability Belongs. It is a diverse, disability-led non-profit that works to create systemic change in how society views and values people with disabilities, and its online resources—such as webinars, training, and consulting—are available to everyone. For those specifically in the disability community, another resource is the 10% ("ten percent") app, founded by Erin Field. It is a newly launched social networking and community-building platform offering tools and opportunities to connect with others who share similar experiences.

- Impact of Environment Size: Smaller workplaces and environments often adapt more easily to allergy accommodations, likely due to fewer bureaucratic hurdles and closer personal relationships. While challenges can still arise, this has been my general experience over decades of navigating accommodations, though inclusive non-profits sometimes differ. This isn't a blanket generalization, just an observation.

9

NON-FOOD PRODUCTS

Reading Non-Food Product Labels

This chapter investigates the often-overlooked world of non-food items where allergens can hide without warning or clear labeling. I've often stood in a store aisle, turning a product over in my hands, scanning the label. It'll say something like "96% natural ingredients," and I'll wonder—*what's in the other 4%?* If you haven't noticed this before, try looking next time you shop. You might be surprised by how vague it is.

At first glance, it might seem harmless. But that lack of transparency can be dangerous when the unidentified ingredients contain allergens. I didn't fully grasp how risky this could be until later in life, when I started looking more closely. The labeling standards for what we put on our skin, use in our homes, or rub near our eyes are shockingly loose compared to food—and for those with life-threatening allergies, the consequences can be severe.

When shopping for products, I typically buy in-store after carefully scanning the ingredient list. If a product claims to be "allergy-friendly" or appears free of my allergens but doesn't clearly state it, I usually use my phone to check if the brand has an online explainer or FAQ for allergen information while still in the store.

If I can't determine the safety of a product within a few minutes, I take photos of the ingredient panels and barcodes of a few promising items and contact the manufacturers once I get home. I also shop for non-food products online, reviewing ingredients panels during the process, but when the product arrives, I make sure it matches what I saw when I bought it. This method is time-consuming, but it's essential for my safety, and it mirrors my food-buying process in many ways because these products could come into contact with my skin or even enter my mouth.

Unfortunately, this is the reality of shopping for food and non-food items with a food allergy. Once I've identified some safe go-to products and brands, shopping becomes much more manageable. Trader Joe's is often a reliable option if I struggle to find a specific product, such as a supplement, beverage, household cleaner, or beauty product. Their product line is helpful, as customers can inquire about allergens in their products and facilities for food and non-food products as long as they're the Trader Joe's brand. Here's a quick recap of my shopping process:

- Check Ingredients In-Store: When shopping, I first study the ingredient panel in-store and in person.

- Verify Online: If a product seems safe for me but isn't 100% clear, I will look up the brand's FAQ on their website from my phone while in the store.

- Contact Later: If I can't determine safety quickly, I take photos of the ingredients panels and barcodes to contact the manufacturer once I get home.

- Shop Online: I also review ingredient panels and order products online, ensuring they match what I saw when they arrived.

When navigating non-food products, allergen safety can feel even more opaque than with food items. Over time, I've developed a strategy to mitigate this uncertainty while staying as informed as possible. Here's a short explainer to reading non-food labels for allergens:

- Check Ingredients: Look for any obvious allergens you know you react to.

- Chemical Names: Familiarize yourself with the chemical, Latin, and scientific names of any allergens you manage or shop for.

- Contact Manufacturer: If needed, contact the manufacturer via email or phone for detailed ingredient information.

Unfortunately, they aren't required to answer or give it to you, but you can always try.

- Patch Test: Before using a new skincare product, you can apply a small amount of the skincare product to a discreet area, such as the forearm or the back of the neck behind the ear, and wait 24 to 48 hours to check for any signs of irritation. You can do this at home if you're comfortable. For more thorough testing, a dermatologist, and in some cases, an allergist can perform clinical patch testing for reactions to specific ingredients or chemicals.

- Household Cleaning Products: When you have environmental, chemical, or food allergies, it's important to exercise caution with cleaning products, as they often lack complete ingredient lists. For those sensitive to fragrances or who have asthma or eczema, like me, it's best to look for products labeled as "fragrance-free" "for sensitive skin" and "dye-free" while also knowing you need to cross-check the ingredients to make sure these claims are accurate.

- Makeup & Skincare: If you have chemical allergies or are attentive to common allergens like lanolin, mica, and various preservatives, finding trustworthy cosmetics and skincare for delicate areas like your face can be tricky. Much like with household products, makeup often lacks a complete ingredient list. When this happens, I find it helpful to email the manufacturer for more information. In terms of reliable seals of approval, you can look for the "National Eczema Association," which requires adhering to strict standards in order to be accepted, and "USDA Organic," which must meet specific farming and ingredient standards.

- Consult Healthcare Provider: If you are unsure about potential allergens, always consult with a healthcare provider, such as your doctor, or ask a pharmacist at your local pharmacy.

I aim to use products with the most limited ingredient lists whenever possible, applying this approach to all non-food items. It's simply easier to understand what's in them. The more familiar I am with the ingredients and the shorter the ingredient list, the better I can ensure my safety and be reaction-free.

Regulations for Non-Food Products

In the US, allergen labeling regulations for non-food products—think toothpaste, soaps, dish soap, laundry detergent, air fresheners, insect repellents, pet grooming products, household cleaners, makeup, hair dye, shampoos, conditioners, and personal care items like deodorants and moisturizers—are even more lax than those for food products (and we already know our food labeling isn't exactly a gold standard).

This means non-food product labeling is even less regulated, despite these items coming into contact with our skin and sometimes even ending up inside our bodies through aerosols and the like. Additionally, allergen labeling rules for alcoholic beverages differ from those for non-alcoholic drinks and other food products. In this section, we'll unpack the current regulations and what they mean for those needing to understand allergen safety.

Please note that I'm not an expert in legalities, but as a food-allergic adult relying on this information, I've done my best to provide accurate details and citations. For deeper insights or specific questions, consult your allergist and explore further. Now, let's dive into cosmetics and personal care products.

Cosmetics and Personal Care Products

Several key regulations guide labeling and safety regarding cosmetics and personal care products. Here's a breakdown of the primary laws and what they mean for allergen labeling:

Food, Drug, and Cosmetic Act (FDCA)

- FDA Oversight: The FDA ensures the safety of cosmetics and personal care products. It defines safety based on its ability to be used without causing harm, supported by scientific evidence and adherence to legal standards. Manufacturers are primarily responsible for ensuring safety, with the FDA providing oversight through regulations, monitoring, and enforcement actions.

- Ingredient Listing: All ingredients must be listed on product labels in descending order of predominance. However, "natural flavors" and "natural fragrances" can contain multiple ingredients, including potential allergens, and specific components are not required to be disclosed.

- Natural Oils and Vegetable Oil: These ingredients should be listed by specific names, but the source might be unclear.

- Fair Packaging and Labeling Act (FPLA): Products must be labeled so consumers can easily identify what the product is, who made it, and how much it contains. Labels must clearly show the product name or type, the name and location of the manufacturer, packer, or distributor, and the net quantity of contents expressed in weight, volume, or count using both metric and U.S. customary units. Accurate labeling provides transparency, but unlike food products, ingredients that may trigger reactions are not always in plain language, which can affect consumers managing allergies, dietary restrictions, or other health concerns.

Allergen Labeling

- Ingredient Disclosure: Allergens like walnut shells or almond oil must be listed by their Latin/scientific names (e.g., "*Juglans regia* (walnut) shell powder," "*Prunus amygdalus dulcis* (sweet almond) oil").

- No Special Formatting: Allergens are not required to be bolded or highlighted.

Navigating Cosmetics and Personal Care Products

When navigating cosmetics and personal care products, I've found it helpful to utilize online resources designed to filter items based on specific allergens. Websites and apps that offer these tools can significantly streamline the search for safer options, especially when the ingredient lists feel overwhelming or inconsistent.

It's also important to be wary of the term hypoallergenic. Because this label isn't regulated or clearly defined, it doesn't guarantee that a product will be allergen-friendly for everyone. For example, I've had skin allergic reactions, like hives, to lanolin and propolis (beeswax), both of which frequently appear in products marketed as hypoallergenic but are problematic allergens for me. In practice, the term often functions more as a marketing strategy than a meaningful safety assurance. Products labeled "fragrance-free" can be somewhat more useful, but even then, reading the full ingredient list remains the safest approach.

Practical Tips for Common Products

- Lip Balm: If you have fruit or nut allergies, you may want to check with the manufacturer to confirm the ingredients in their "natural flavors," as these can sometimes contain these allergens.

- Fragrances: Investigate the specific components of "natural fragrances" to ensure they don't include allergens or irritants that might affect you. This applies to perfumes, too! As someone with a lanolin allergy, I've learned that many fragrances in shampoos, soaps, and perfumes are often lanolin-based without specifying.

- Moisturizers & Hand Soaps: If you're allergic to certain oils—like sweet almond or sesame—check carefully to confirm whether those oils are used. Milk and milk-derived ingredients also appear frequently in these products, yet they're often unclear or undisclosed. In many shared spaces—stores, hotels, workplaces, hospitals—that level of detail isn't accessible, so extra caution is needed with unlabeled items.

Finding What Works for You

By keeping these pointers in mind, you can better navigate the complexities of cosmetic and personal care labeling. Improved labeling laws are needed to protect consumers, as airborne and topical allergens can still pose serious health risks and are often inadequately labeled.

I prefer using ingredients and products from brands that have told me there are no peanuts used in their facilities, but comfort levels with these practices may vary—choose what works best for you. For my skincare routine, lighter oils like coconut, jojoba, argan, and rosehip are my go-to during summer, while heavier oils such as sesame, sweet almond, and avocado provide better hydration in winter or for extremely dry skin. I use these oils on my face and body and have enjoyed the nourishing results for years. Growing up with Ayurvedic practices, this approach feels natural and comforting.

You can use plain oils or infuse them with fresh ingredients for added benefits. If you make blends with fresh items, keep the amounts small to prevent spoilage. A minimalist routine works well for me and my ultra dry skin. I like pairing oils with fragrance-free lotions like Vanicream and Yobee Skin (Dr. Ruchi Gupta's brand, which I've come to swear by) with single-ingredient oils that avoid my allergen. I find that for my dry skin, using an oil first, and a cream or lotion second on top, works well for me to seal the moisture in. Of course, everyone's skin and skincare routines are different and need to be adapted accordingly.

Household Cleaners & Detergents

Did you know that allergen labeling rules for household products like cleaners and detergents are vastly different from food labeling, too? This can make it tricky to determine which products are truly safe. Regulations play a key role in what information is (and isn't) disclosed on these products, so understanding them is essential for making safer choices, especially if you manage allergies or sensitivities. Here's a deeper look at how these rules shape allergen safety and tips for navigating the shelves with greater confidence.

Federal Hazardous Substances Act (FHSA)

Under this act, the CPSC (Consumer Product Safety Commission) regulates hazardous household substances, including cleaners. Products must have appropriate warnings if they pose hazards like toxicity, flammability, or the apparent potential to cause allergic reactions. However, since anyone can react to anything, this isn't extensive, and I imagine it only covers common allergens.

Labeling of Hazardous Art Materials Act (LHAMA)

The LHAMA primarily ensures that art materials, which may contain potentially hazardous substances, are labeled with appropriate warnings to safeguard users. This act mandates that manufacturers test their products for chronic health hazards and provide clear labeling based on the findings. However, LHAMA focuses on hazards such as toxicity, carcinogenicity, and reproductive harm rather than allergic reactions. While anaphylaxis is indeed a severe and potentially life-threatening allergic reaction, LHAMA does not explicitly address allergens in its definition of hazardous materials. As a result, products that may cause allergic reactions, including anaphylaxis, are not necessarily covered under LHAMA's labeling requirements.

It is very important for individuals with anaphylactic allergies to read all product labels carefully and be aware of potential allergens, even if they are not highlighted as hazardous under LHAMA. This includes checking for common allergens such as peanuts, tree nuts, milk, eggs, fish, shellfish, soy, wheat, sesame, and others, even in art materials that their labeling might not cover. Products like play-dough, glue, and other craft supplies often contain wheat or other top allergens, such as corn, posing a risk for individuals with food allergies.

Environmental Protection Agency (EPA)

Under FIFRA, the EPA regulates products that contain antimicrobial or pesticidal properties. These products are only required to disclose active ingredients and potential risks. This lack of transparency can frustrate consumers, particularly those with allergies who need to know if a product contains substances they are sensitive to or life-threateningly allergic to. To navigate this issue, individuals can contact the manufacturer directly for detailed ingredient information. Additionally, exploring alternative products labeled with specific allergen information or opting to make their own "safe" versions may help mitigate risks. Proactively researching and verifying product ingredients ensures informed choices and promotes safer product usage for individuals with allergies. For those interested in alternative solutions, making homemade household products with limited ingredients can provide control over allergen exposure.

Key Considerations for Non-Food Allergen Disclosure

Understanding the complexities of allergen labeling in cosmetics and other non-food products can empower consumers to make safer choices. Here's a breakdown of the essential details:

- Fragrance Allergens: In the United States, manufacturers are not required to disclose individual fragrance allergens, such as limonene or linalool, on cosmetic product labels, regardless of their concentration. The FDA mandates that "fragrance" or "perfume" be listed as an ingredient but without the need to specify the individual components that make up the fragrance. This need for more transparency can be problematic for consumers with sensitivities or allergies to specific fragrance ingredients.

- Dye Allergens: Similarly, dyes used in cosmetics and personal care products are typically listed by their chemical names or Color Index (CI) numbers, which may not be easily recognizable to the average consumer. While the FDA requires that color additives used in cosmetics be approved for safety, there's no mandatory labeling specifically highlighting potential allergens within these dyes. This can pose challenges for individuals with sensitivities or allergies to certain colorants, especially since these ingredients are often listed in a way that may not indicate their allergenic potential.

- Food-Derived Allergens in Cosmetics: In the United States, the Fair Packaging and Labeling Act (FPLA) requires cosmetic products, personal care items, and other non-food products sold at retail to list all ingredients, and this requirement is enforced by the FDA. However, some ingredients that may trigger allergic reactions, including those derived from common allergenic sources, can appear under technical or chemical names that do not clearly indicate their origin—for example, an almond-derived ingredient may not be readily recognizable as a tree nut. Because the ingredients are not required to be highlighted in plain language, consumers with allergies may have difficulty identifying potential triggers.

- Comparison to the European Union: In contrast, the European Union (EU) has stricter regulations regarding labeling potential allergens in cosmetics, including allergenic fragrances and dyes. For example, in the EU, fragrance allergens like limonene or linalool must be listed on the product label if they exceed 0.001% in leave-on products or 0.01% in rinse-off products. Similarly, certain colorants that are known allergens must also be clearly identified on labels, providing consumers with more detailed information to help them avoid allergens.

- Labeling Terms, Certifications, and "Free From" Claims: Terms like "fragrance-free" or "dye-free" must be truthful. Misleading claims can lead to action from regulatory bodies like the FDA or FTC. For example, a product labeled as "fragrance-free" must not contain any fragrance ingredients, while "dye-free" products should not contain color additives. As mentioned, the term "hypoallergenic" and many other marketing terms remains unregulated in the US, meaning that products labeled as such are not required to meet any specific criteria and may still contain ingredients that cause allergic reactions in some individuals. Alternatively, other countries have regulations requiring dermatological testing, scientific data, or clinical studies to substantiate such claims and ensure consumer safety.

Understanding Industry Standards

While federal regulations set the baseline for safety and labeling, industry-driven standards also significantly shape practices within the cosmetics industry. These voluntary programs and organizations contribute to the oversight of cosmetic products, though they are not substitutes for mandatory regulations. Understanding these standards can provide additional context for how products are reviewed and labeled:

Cosmetic Ingredient Review (CIR)

An industry-sponsored organization that reviews the safety of cosmetic ingredients. While the CIR's recommendations can influence labeling practices, participation is voluntary, and its guidelines do not carry the same weight as federal regulations.

Voluntary Cosmetic Registration Program (VCRP)

A program where manufacturers can voluntarily register their cosmetic products and ingredients with the FDA. While it promotes greater transparency, it is worth noting that this registration is not required by law, and therefore, not all products on the market are registered.

These above details are drawn from the relevant US regulatory frameworks I investigated, reflecting the current requirements and practices for labeling non-food products. I hope to see changes in these legislative policies to demand that companies take more responsibility for protecting consumers with allergies. Enhanced labeling standards and definitions for vague terms like "hypoallergenic" could significantly reduce the risk for those with severe allergic reactions and improve consumer safety.

Alcohol Labeling Laws

As I mentioned before, alcoholic beverages aren't held to the same standards. Currently, the Treasury Department's TTB Division, responsible for regulating alcohol labeling, does not require the disclosure of the top 9 allergens. However, there is ongoing advocacy and collaboration among organizations to push for this change at the federal level.

By the time this book is released, I'm hopeful that alcoholic beverage labeling will be more consistently enforced and transparent, bringing us closer to a future where these products are held to clearer standards. But with ongoing FDA budget cuts and the stance of the current government administration, I'm trying to manage my expectations. People with both common and less common allergies that fall outside the top 9 allergens should all be careful when consuming alcohol. It's important to check what the beverage is derived from. For example, amaretto is made from almonds, vodka can be made from wheat, corn, potatoes, or even grapes, and bourbon is typically made from corn, often blended with rye, wheat, or barley. Liqueurs and flavored spirits may also contain ingredients like dairy, wheat, or tree nuts, and some cocktails use egg whites to create foam.

Because labeling is not required or complete, I recommend contacting the manufacturers directly and reviewing their websites for full ingredient information and potential allergen risks. I've often felt overwhelmed at breweries or bars, unsure if the environment is safe, but I do my best to try to find out as much information as possible to understand the risk-level I'm taking. Ciders are often suggested as a gluten-free alternative to beer, but it's still important to check labels or contact the manufacturer, as some may contain added flavors or ingredients that could pose risks for those with food allergies.

Often, I opt not to order alcoholic drinks and bring my own water bottle and a KN95 mask to avoid any peanut contamination. If I trust the space but am unfamiliar with their offerings, I might stick to a simple soda water with lime and ask them to rinse the glass extra before serving and possibly skip the ice (which can often be contaminated). It's important to do what feels best to enjoy yourself in the moment. A friendly reminder: even mocktail ingredients can be misleading and sneaky, so checking for potential allergens is always wise.

A Word on Delta-9, Drugs, and Marijuana Products

Products like marijuana edibles, THC and CBD beverages, gummies, and vapes are not classified as "food" by the FDA, which means they are exempt from the food labeling laws that help protect people with allergic diseases. This lack of regulation can create serious gaps in transparency and safety. I approach these products with the same level of scrutiny as I do food and alcohol—asking questions, researching ingredients, and reaching out to manufacturers when needed. Because of this, I tend to stick to a few trusted brands that have been responsive and informed about allergens and cross-contact.

Personally, I've welcomed the growing regulation of marijuana products, as it offers me a greater sense of security knowing they're less likely to be laced, more likely to be stored and produced in clean, traceable facilities, and that there's a better chance of accountability if something goes wrong or gets contaminated by allergens. For anyone with food allergies, it's important to treat these products with the same level of caution and awareness as anything else you might consume.

Impaired Judgment & Allergy Risk: Alcohol, Delta-9, and Other Substances

One often overlooked issue with alcohol and marijuana products—whether Delta-9, edibles, or other drugs—is how they lower our inhibitions and impair judgment. For someone with food allergies, this can be incredibly dangerous. Alcohol, for example, not only makes it harder to think clearly, but it may also intensify the severity of a reaction through what's known in allergy science as an augmentation factor—meaning it can worsen symptoms that might otherwise be milder.

When under the influence, you might forget to check labels, eat something you normally wouldn't, or misplace your epinephrine. You could also be too impaired to recognize early symptoms of a reaction or too slow to respond. I can't tell you how many times I've had a Delta-9 or marijuana product and spiraled into anxiety, unsure if I was experiencing a real reaction or just hyper-fixating on normal mouth sensations because I was high. These are real risks to consider. Any substance that alters your awareness or delays your ability to act deserves extra caution when you're managing an anaphylactic food allergy.

That's not to say you need to avoid these substances; I don't, but it's essential to have a plan, stay prepared, and surround yourself with people who understand your allergies and know what to do in an emergency. Communication with others and having clarity for yourself is key, especially before alcohol or drugs have a chance to cloud it.

The Peanut Butter Lush Soap

Lush, known for its high-quality handmade cosmetics, has always stood out as a brand committed to using natural, vegetarian, and cruelty-free ingredients. As someone who's been a lifelong vegetarian and a passionate advocate for animal rights, Lush aligns perfectly with my values. My journey volunteering with PETA began when I was just 10 years old, reflecting a dedication to ending animal cruelty that has stayed with me ever since.

In high school, I had a friend who was a big fan of Lush products. She often used them, and I always admired how wonderful they smelled. Eventually, she even started working at Lush, and I remember thinking it would be a dream to work there someday. Despite my admiration for the brand, I've always been sensitive to fragrances. This sensitivity ultimately led me to reconsider working there, as I knew it might not be the best environment for me, even though it was a place I greatly respected and aligned with on so many levels.

Fast-forward many years to when I was engaged and planning my wedding. I wanted to create special gift bags for my bridesmaids and close friends. Naturally, Lush came to mind as the perfect place to find thoughtful, unique gifts I felt good about buying. I went in-store and carefully selected glittery, swirly soaps and beautifully scented bath bombs, each one chosen with a particular person in mind. After checking out, I started thinking that maybe my fiancé would also appreciate some gifts for his groomsmen.

After paying for my items, I strolled over to the hand lotion area and began exploring the different scents. Thankfully, I didn't touch, smell, or try any samples, as I had done earlier with cautious curiosity—never expecting to see "peanuts" listed as an ingredient in anything there.

But then, I spotted a hand lotion that made me double-take. There was nothing bold or distinct to set it apart from the other scents, but I luckily caught a glimpse of the words "peanut butter" on the label, written in small, easily overlooked font. As I read further, I discovered that the lotion was made from nut butters, including peanut and cashew butter. I was floored.

Panic surged through my chest as I bolted out of the store, heading straight to the nearby mall bathroom to wash my hands. Even holding my bag of purchases, I couldn't stop wondering, "Did the person who checked me out use that hand cream? Am I contaminated with peanut butter?" I closely monitored myself for symptoms, hearing my fast pulse thudding in my ears, keeping my epinephrine at the ready, but the fear lingered, leaving me in a state of anxiety.

I felt incredibly lucky that I hadn't touched that lotion or experienced any allergic reaction just from being in the store. The risk of cross-contact seemed high, with people trying products and samples from the open jars left and right. I couldn't believe this lotion wasn't marked with an eye-catching warning for those with life-threatening nut allergies. Even a small sign saying, "Beware: Allergen Alert! This Lotion Contains Nut Ingredients," wouldn't have seemed like a stretch to include. This incident made me question what other allergens they might be using, so I meticulously combed through their website, zooming in on every ingredient list and piece of allergen content I could find.

After reaching out to Lush to express my concerns, I received a detailed response that shed some light on their approach to allergens in their products. Their response emphasized that severe allergic reactions are something they strive to avoid. They mentioned that, while peanuts are a common allergen and usually avoided in their products, the hand lotion I mentioned does contain organic peanut and cashew butter. They also directed me to their online LUSHopedia, which provides detailed information on ingredients, although the UK version offers even more comprehensive details.

And there you have it. I haven't shopped at Lush since. Even though I love their mission and the products I've used in the past, it's not worth it. I made sure to reply to them about how surprised I was and how dangerous it is. Once I started my *Invisibly Allergic* Blog, I included this information about their products to beware of on my website to raise awareness about needing to look out for literal nut butters and the top 9 allergen ingredients in non-food products.

Even after my kindly worded response, it's been over 9 years since this happened, and a recent check of their website shows that they still offer the same peanut butter and cashew butter hand lotion.

This underscores the urgent need for clear and comprehensive allergen labeling for food and all types of products. Allergens in personal care items can pose sobering risks, and the current lack of stringent regulations and mandatory disclosures in non-food categories creates a significant gap in consumer safety. It's imperative that all brands, not just Lush, take proactive measures to protect their customers by providing transparent and prominent allergen information. This won't happen independently without legislation requiring it.

As the prevalence of allergies continues to rise, comprehensive labeling becomes increasingly essential. I am deeply committed to advancing this cause but can't do it alone. If you share this passion for change, have legal experience, or know someone who does, connect with me through the contact form on my *Invisibly Allergic* website. Your support and insights can help drive meaningful change in allergen safety and labeling practices.

Closing Thoughts & Additional Context

- Non-Food Products: Before using non-food products, especially those that come into contact with my mouth—like lipsticks, lip moisturizers, or items such as herbal supplements, vitamins, and tea—I follow the same process when checking ingredients in food. I will contact the manufacturer to inquire if peanuts are processed in the same facility, and I adopted this practice after discovering that some vitamins, teas, and lotions I used were produced and packaged on equipment shared with peanuts. I also include the Latin name of the allergen in my inquiries if it seems relevant.

- Transparency Issues: Non-food products, such as personal care items and household cleaners, often lack clear and consistent allergen labeling. This gap in labeling practices poses considerable risks for individuals with allergies. Unlike food products, which are subject to stricter labeling requirements, many non-food items do not have to disclose individual allergen components, leaving consumers vulnerable to accidental exposure. The absence of comprehensive regulations means that even products containing known allergens can go unmarked, making it challenging to make informed and safe choices.

- Shopping Strategy: When shopping for non-food items, always examine the in-store and online ingredient panels. If you need to, you can inquire to verify allergen information through the brand's website or by contacting the manufacturer directly. If you can't confirm safety in-store, take photos of product labels and barcodes to follow up later. Despite the convenience of online shopping, ensure the product received matches the expected allergen information.

- Latin, Scientific, and Chemical Names: For effective allergen management, be familiar with the scientific names, Latin names, and chemical names of your known allergens. Instead of memorizing them, write them down or save them in a Notes section of your phone for cross-reference.

- Trader Joe's: Recommended for their detailed allergen

information on food and non-food items. You can call their phone product line while shopping to find out more information about allergens in products and facilities. You provide them with the barcode of each item, and they will research that specific facility and let you know the details.

- DIY Solutions: Creating limited-ingredient products for skincare and household use has been liberating and cost-effective. It gives me complete control over what goes into these products, providing reassurance and peace of mind by ensuring they are free from unwanted allergens and irritants. This hands-on approach saves money and guarantees that I know exactly what I'm using in my daily routines.

10

MEDIA'S IMPACT ON FOOD ALLERGY AWARENESS

Evolution of Food Allergy Portrayals in Media

In a world where media shapes our understanding of health and safety, food allergies are often depicted as a dramatic subplot or a laughable condition in mainstream movies, television, commercials, and social media content. Have you ever found yourself cringing at an exaggerated portrayal of a condition you know shouldn't be the punchline of a joke? Perhaps you've encountered a misrepresentation of a disability or health issue, LGBTQ+ identities, transgender experiences, deafness, blindness, mental health conditions, chronic illnesses, or neurodiversity in a way that feels dismissive or harmful. Food allergies are no exception. Media portrayals can be a double-edged sword—capable of raising awareness and fostering empathy, yet also prone to spreading myths and reinforcing negative stereotypes.

This chapter delves into how food allergies are depicted across various media platforms, shedding light on both the beneficial and harmful impacts these portrayals have on public perception, from the moments of genuine insight to the all-too-common dangerous inaccuracies of anaphylaxis.

Since the late 20th century (yes, it makes me feel a bit nostalgic and old), especially from 1985 to 1999 (which, okay, does predate me a little), there has been a notable rise in reported food allergy cases and, with it, growing public awareness. Yet, during this early period and into the 2000s, up until around the mid-2010s, media portrayals often grossly missed the mark, lacking accuracy and sensitivity to this condition. Instead of sharing helpful information to promote understanding, these depictions perpetuated incorrect stereotypes and spread misinformation about the seriousness. Food allergies are not a mere lifestyle choice or preference—they are a potentially deadly condition that can lead to both physical and mental health challenges, often daily.

Early media portrayals of food allergies often sensationalized allergic reactions, particularly anaphylaxis. These depictions exaggerated the drama and presented the reactions as intense events that instantaneously resolved almost as quickly as they appeared. Such portrayals led to misunderstandings about the actual life-or-death reality and symptoms of food allergies, including how to properly handle and treat them.

There is a social media account I follow of a board-certified allergist who often debunks these types of extreme portrayals, such as people purposefully eating their allergens on TikTok for shock value. While I appreciate his content and its variety beyond debunking videos, it's disheartening to see how much allergy mockery and other inappropriate material there is for him to tackle.

In reality, anaphylaxis is typically terrifying for the person experiencing it. The immune system goes into full fight-or-flight mode, and the situation demands immediate action. This means administering an epinephrine injector in the correct spot—usually the upper thigh—and calling for emergency medical help right away. You may also need to monitor the person closely and, in some cases, use more than one dose of epinephrine. Something I've never seen shown in these dramatic media allergic reaction portrayals is that it's advised to lay the person down to aid blood flow to the heart and to prepare for the possibility of unconsciousness. Unfortunately, these critical life-saving aspects are repeatedly absent in representations, like the basics of carrying and using epinephrine promptly to ensure it can save the person's life.

While social media platforms and well-connected food allergy non-profits can often advocate for quickly removing inaccurate content, it remains puzzling why such portrayals are approved in the first place. It sounds obvious, but I wish people wouldn't share content that may influence others to try to eat their known allergens. I'd have hoped by now the media would look to people living the allergy experience to get advice on providing firsthand accounts and giving accurate leadership direction. These resources are valuable and should be more widely used.

This issue extends beyond food allergy and allergic disease misrepresentations and includes inaccurate portrayals of various health conditions, disabilities, and marginalized identities, as well as harmful and offensive messaging.

Accurate depictions are crucial for educating the public and showcasing legislation that benefits the communities depicted. Regarding food allergies, proper media representation can significantly impact emergency responses and broader advocacy efforts, making a real difference in how food allergies are understood and managed.

On a related note, it's exciting to see new advancements in epinephrine delivery methods in the media. As I've said, the Neffy nasal-spray epinephrine—AKA the first FDA-approved needle-free alternative—is officially available. Hopefully, Aquestive's Anaphylm, the under-the-tongue epinephrine, isn't far behind. This is hugely encouraging for the food allergy community, as needle-free options can help reduce fear and make life-saving treatment more accessible.

For the past few years, I've used the epinephrine brand Auvi-Q, an injector with an audio component that provides step-by-step medication administration instructions. This feature has been life-changing for me, offering more clarity and ease for the user and those assisting in an emergency. Imagine how impactful it could be if the media accurately showcased these super cool advancements and provided realistic portrayals of food allergies instead.

To encourage this, I offer media consulting services on my

website and put in extra effort to try and make it easy for anyone interested to find if searched for online. These types of resources are available for most types of representation and ready to help improve the accuracy of portrayals across the board. Plus, it gets money directly into the hands of those living the experience the media is wanting to represent.

When I talk about a fanatical reaction, many of us are probably picturing the same scene from the 2005 movie *Hitch*, where Will Smith's character suffers an anaphylactic reaction to shellfish. The scene shows his face swelling dramatically and comically (though I never found it funny). While it might've aimed to highlight the seriousness of allergies with a touch of humor, it completely misrepresents the reality. If the character were genuinely experiencing that much facial and esophagus swelling, he would be physically unable to talk through it. When I experienced these symptoms, I was dizzy, losing my vision, losing my hearing, and going unconscious.

The worst part to me is that the plot neglects to show the necessary administration of potentially life-saving epinephrine, which someone with an IgE-mediated food allergy should ideally be carrying on them, as it is the only way to reverse his symptoms. The movie doesn't show the steps of calling 911 and going to a hospital, either, actions that would be necessary in such a reaction. This is just one example that is commonly referenced. Not to mention, he self-medicates with antihistamines, which would not be able to treat his reaction and would also not be advised by the medical field, as they can hide symptoms of a more severe allergic reaction.

Annoyingly, two new movies released in September 2025—*The Roses* and *Freakier Friday*—both use scenes like this. What are the odds they'd even be in theaters at the same time? I literally walked past *The Roses*, told my friends why I wasn't seeing it (after people in the allergy community warned it was especially triggering, and because I didn't feel like supporting it with my dollars), and then went to *Freakier Friday*—only to sit through something similar. That one blindsided me with not one but five food allergy jokes I counted, including one eerily similar to the *Hitch* scene. Super unoriginal. I'm not impressed. Why is this still happening? Anyway, I digress.

Recognizing these inaccuracies makes it even more meaningful when progress is made in food allergy representation—and it motivates us to keep pushing for further improvements. In fact, a new film, *May Contain: My Life*, is about to be released that I was lucky enough to preview, and it still gives me goosebumps just thinking about it. This is a must-watch. It takes us inside the life-or-death reality of food allergies, where every day is a balancing act between survival and simply trying to fit in. The film highlights the relentless challenges faced by over 30 million Americans living with this condition. Watch the trailer, share it, and join in on the movement to make food allergy awareness, safety, and inclusion standard in every space.

Over the past 15 years, advocacy, medical advancements, and increased awareness have brought more nuanced and accurate portrayals of food allergies in the media, or at least encouraged efforts to remove offensive material. I'm happy to see these strides.

The Power of Large Platforms & Social Media's Role

While acknowledging progress made in food allergy representation, addressing ongoing issues is pivotal. In 2024, a Super Bowl commercial from Uber Eats previewed a scene that made light of life-threatening food allergies, strikingly similar to the 2005 *Hitch* portrayal (talk about unoriginal!). The public preview quickly drew backlash from the food allergy community, including myself, across TikTok and Instagram. Advocacy efforts succeeded, and Uber Eats removed the offending scene before the commercial officially aired, highlighting how powerful collective action can be in protecting accurate and respectful representation.

The response was swift and unified by the food allergy community. Our efforts were successful: UberEats altered the advertisement, ensuring that the problematic content did not air during the Super Bowl, which approximately 112 million viewers watched. This collective action prevented the dissemination of potentially harmful messages about food allergies to a massive audience. Today, while challenges remain, there is an emphasis on accurate representation and the potential impact of media portrayals on public understanding and empathy toward food allergy sufferers.

The power of large media platforms is evident in this incident, showcasing how a single commercial from a major brand can significantly influence the lives of over 33 million people with food allergies and their social circles. Large brands and corporations are especially responsible for the use of their platforms. For them to leverage their influence for good, avoiding spreading harmful or misleading information about any community is essential. Promoting bullying or mocking individuals based on their health conditions, disabilities, or identities is simply unacceptable.

The words and actions of these powerful entities can profoundly impact mental health, shaping public perceptions and either fostering understanding or perpetuating negative stigma. Ensuring accurate, respectful representation is essential to prevent harm and benefit the well-being of all individuals. Mental health, a critical aspect of overall health influenced by these dynamics, will be the next topic I explore in-depth in the next chapter.

Just a few months following the Super Bowl incident, another controversy arose involving a Snickers commercial promoting in-flight sales, saying, "it's not flying without peanuts," despite well-known and publicized ongoing efforts by the food allergy community to secure better accommodations for air travelers. This commercial sparked outrage for seemingly disregarding the risks posed to those with nut allergies on airplanes.

The connection between peanuts and air travel originated in the early days of commercial aviation when peanuts were offered as a low-cost, shelf-stable snack. The phrase "as cheap as peanuts" was part of airline marketing in the mid-20th century, reinforcing the affordability of both the flights and the snack. Over time, peanuts became associated with flying and served routinely. What started as a convenient, inexpensive offering eventually became part of airline culture. So much so that the peanut industry began to rely on the exposure and product demand generated through commercial aviation.

This incident underscores the community's continuing challenges in advocating for greater awareness and safety measures, particularly in high-profile media like commercial advertising. Even with petitions and some progress on airline accommodations, commercials like this reveal a persistent ignorance of the life-threatening nature of food allergies. The fact that such commercials can still be produced and aired despite recent and similar controversies highlights the significant work needed to educate the public about the dangers of trivializing food allergies in media portrayals. Some in the food allergy community speculate that these types of publicity stunts are designed to attract press, Instagram tags, and traffic, and I sincerely hope that's not the case.

A recent comment that struck a chord with me was made by Charli D'Amelio, a TikTok star who rose to fame for her dance videos and later became a reality TV personality. I'd been seeing her videos on my Instagram and thought I'd try watching her reality show. Well, just a few minutes into the very first episode of *The D'Amelio Show*, titled "Charli D'Amelio? What the Heck?" Charli made a comment, stating she "would rather die than have a food allergy." I felt a heavy pang in my heart and paused the show, ultimately deciding not to continue watching. Given that the show reaches millions, Charli's influence is undeniable; even I, someone not in her target audience, was drawn in and influenced online to watch the show. It turns out that she's among the top 5 influencers on social media in the world, with over 155.5 million followers.

Therefore, it was incredibly disheartening that such a comment wasn't flagged as offensive by editors or the production team on their show. Such remarks can profoundly affect the mental health of those with food allergies, making them feel marginalized and devalued. This instance highlights how a large platform can sometimes spread negative messages, underscoring the need for influencers to use their reach responsibly.

As a Bachelor Nation fan—someone who occasionally watches *The Bachelor* and *The Bachelorette*—I was bummed to see a cast bio where one contestant, Devon, commented on his food allergy. His ABC profile listed a "fun fact": "Devon loves eating shrimp tacos despite being allergic to shrimp." Hmm, I thought.

This reminded me, again, of the all-too-common viral videos where people deliberately consume their allergens or pretend to have an allergy. Given the severe and potentially fatal nature of a true IgE allergy to shrimp, seeing such risks downplayed is deeply concerning. Such behavior could be seen as dangerously reckless and might even be interpreted as a form of self-harm. Unfortunately, it was a highly discussed point on all the *Bachelor* podcasts I listened to. Each mention on the *Bachelor* podcasts stung a little sharper, the humor hitting like an accidental slap on a fresh sunburn. Listening to others' laughter about allergies takes a toll on me mentally, and it's something I encounter all too often.

It felt like such a missed opportunity for introspection and understanding, especially since he's part of the food allergy community himself. It's always disappointing when influencers or celebrities with food allergies downplay their experiences and don't include information on how food allergy reactivity is a spectrum and how their experience isn't a one-size-fits-all, applying to the entirety of the food allergy community. Given that the show attracts millions of viewers per episode, the production should have been more responsible by avoiding the perpetuation of the idea that food allergies can be ignored. Instead, they could have included an engaging and genuinely fun "fun fact."

Comments like Charli D'Amelio's and the contestant from *The Bachelorette* undermine the daily challenges faced by those with food allergies and hinder efforts to raise awareness. Whether they mean it to or not, this contributes to a lack of proper accommodation, exacerbating the social and emotional burdens on individuals managing these conditions.

Social media platforms like Facebook, Reddit, Instagram, TikTok, and YouTube have become strong tools for raising awareness about food allergies. These platforms enable individuals to share real-life stories and offer a genuine community, connecting those facing similar experiences. Still, it's essential to recognize that social media can also contribute to mental health challenges—such as comparison, exposure to triggering content, and misinformation. This includes "fake" or misleading content, as well as harmful generalizations like the claim that "food allergies are a fad diet." There's also a tendency for people to confuse correlation with causation, like assuming that eating a specific food once or using a specific product led to developing a condition, when the reality is far more complex. Whether these posts are made with good intentions or not, they can be damaging.

An international reality TV star, Jack Fowler, shared a video of his near-death experience while flying with Emirates Airlines in June 2024, and it has continued to horrify many. He had the foresight to film his experience of continually being reassured that his on-flight meal was free of his allergen, cashews, and yet, the meal had cashews in it.

On camera, you can see him experiencing a very vulnerable,

life-threatening reaction, looking unwell and out of it, injecting himself with his epinephrine in the airplane bathroom with his pants down. He later shared that he required five tanks of oxygen until he was able to get rushed to a hospital on the ground. It's an experience no one should go through, much less have to document so publicly for people to take it seriously. Yet, that's the reality for those with food allergies when the wider community doesn't fully understand our conditions.

Natasha's Foundation based in the UK has advocated for better food labeling following their 15-year-old daughter's tragic death from eating a sandwich and suffering an allergic reaction while on a British Airways flight in 2016. Natasha Ednan-Laperouse had a life-threatening allergy to sesame seeds, and before the flight, she purchased a baguette from a Pret-A-Manger store at the Airport. Unbeknownst to her and her family, the baguette contained sesame seeds baked into the dough, which were not clearly labeled on the packaging or able to be visually seen.

Shortly after eating the sandwich, Natasha began experiencing symptoms of an allergic reaction while on board the airplane, including difficulty breathing and hives. Her father, who was traveling with her, administered two EpiPen injections. Yet, despite his efforts and the assistance of the cabin crew and a doctor on board, Natasha's condition continued to worsen. The plane made an emergency landing where she was rushed to a hospital, tragically suffered cardiac arrest, and was pronounced dead later that day.

As I write this, I get emotionally distraught. Whenever I see her family advocating online for food allergy awareness and regulations, I think about how her father was with her and how they were doing everything right, reading the labels and being cautious, yet she couldn't be saved. That's the reality of living with a food allergy; you can go from healthy and thriving to dying in mere moments.

Natasha's death revealed significant issues with the UK food labeling practices at the time, as her allergen was purposefully in the bread but not disclosed in the ingredients. The Pret-A-Manger sandwich did not have a specific allergen label, as the company followed regulations that did not require individual product labeling for on-site items.

Her parents have since become prominent advocates for improved food allergen labeling and safety. Their efforts led to introducing "Natasha's Law" in the UK, which mandates stricter labeling requirements for pre-packaged foods to include a complete list of ingredients and emphasize allergens. This law came into effect in October 2021 and aims to prevent similar tragedies from occurring. I've emailed their organization and followed along with their social media accounts as they continue progressing and raising global awareness. I deeply admire their strength and resilience. At the same time, I want to acknowledge that no one should have to endure the loss of a loved one to something that could be prevented.

There is one more story I need to share about the devastating consequences of anaphylaxis and mislabeling. In January 2024, Órla Baxendale, a young woman from East Lancashire, UK, tragically lost her life after eating a mislabeled cookie in New York City. The packaging failed to disclose the presence of peanuts, a major allergen, in violation of FDA regulations. Although she received an epinephrine injection and was rushed to the hospital, her life could not be saved.

Simply put: if food labeling practices were more thorough, and food allergies handled more seriously in the United States, her death could have been prevented. An investigation revealed that the bakery responsible for the cookie had neglected to comply with FDA labeling requirements, which mandate the clear identification of top allergens like peanuts on food packaging. This mistake directly caused Órla's fatal allergic reaction and underscores the critical need for strict enforcement of food labeling laws to protect those with food allergies.

In the wake of this tragedy, her family has become advocates for stronger regulation and greater awareness of food allergy risks, and they are pursuing legal action against the bakery. However, no lawsuit can bring back their daughter. This case highlights the ongoing need for accurate food labeling in the US and globally to safeguard those with food allergies. It's really for everyone, as an allergy to food can develop in anyone at any time, to any food.

This story deeply resonated with me, especially after having traveled to Ireland (Republic of Ireland) and experienced their food labeling laws firsthand. Ireland follows the European Union's food labeling regulations, which I discussed in Chapter 6.

I can't help but think about how Órla likely trusted food labels in a way that's far less reliable here in the US. The contrast is heartbreaking and still devastates me to this day. Knowing that I could shop for food in stores and dine out considerably more safely in Ireland and across the EU was eye opening for me. Even with Brexit occurring in 2020, the UK made up of England, Scotland, Wales, and Northern Ireland, it appears the UK still follows more of the EU rules to avoid a hard border with the remaining EU. I believe those traveling to the US aren't aware of the lack of comprehensive labeling protections in the US, and misleading labels, and this isn't discussed enough on a global scale.

As soon as I returned from my trip abroad, I frantically emailed the FARE advocacy team asking what we can do here in the US to start getting closer to the EU's labeling laws and practices. This was my first real introduction to US policy, as I don't have a background in law and had yet to attend any events around food policy. I began learning about the realistic landscape I was up against, including the groups likely to oppose state-level food labeling laws in my state of Kentucky—such as restaurant associations or others concerned about increased costs and added regulatory hurdles.

At the time, my advocacy contact at FARE explained the key

differences between the EU and US governments, including why this kind of change would need to happen at the state level rather than federally. There is currently no federal mechanism in Congress to support such a shift, so any change would need to be pursued state by state.

As disappointing as it was to learn that we couldn't simply adopt the EU's food labeling system due to the way the FDA and Congress operate, gaining that understanding was still incredibly valuable. I also learned that it typically takes years for a bill to become law in the US, and that timeline can vary greatly. That said, there are exceptions. The FASTER Act, which added sesame as the ninth major allergen requiring labeling, passed relatively quickly in 2021, giving many of us hope that meaningful change is possible when there's enough momentum and bipartisan support. Still, it's a complex and often slow-moving process.

Amid the growing number of viral news segments aimed at the food allergy community—something I've never experienced on my own news station but often see shared online—one particularly distressing episode from ITV's *This Morning* featuring an interview with Nick Ferrari struck a nerve and has stayed with me.

While I won't delve into quoting the specifics of his callous remarks, Ferrari essentially expressed that he didn't care if people with nut allergies "dropped dead" on airplanes, prioritizing his desire to eat peanuts over their safety. To make matters worse, there was nervous laughter from the newscasters, rather than challenging such harmful views. As someone deeply familiar with the challenges of living with food allergies, witnessing moments like this cuts beyond the surface. They can trigger internal battles with self-worth and belonging: *What's wrong with me? Do I matter?* Navigating these emotional minefields, both in media portrayals and personal interactions, takes an immense toll on mental health.

Misguided jokes or dismissive attitudes in the media can undermine the vigilance necessary for managing this chronic condition. The stakes are real—a bite of the wrong food can trigger a severe allergic reaction, and cross-contact lurks in unsuspecting places, posing constant threats to our health and safety.

Positive Portrayals in Media

In the world of food allergies, every accurate and empathetic portrayal in the media serves as a beacon of hope and understanding. I've seen firsthand how powerful these portrayals can be, especially through commercials and educational materials created by dedicated food allergy organizations like FARE and Food Allergy Canada. These groups, driven by a profound sense of duty, craft messages that resonate with those of us navigating life with food allergies.

I remember stumbling upon a heartfelt blog post by a fellow allergy warrior. Her words vividly captured our daily challenges and triumphs—from meticulously scrutinizing ingredient labels to the anxiety of dining out. Influencers and bloggers like her, by sharing their personal stories, have managed to weave a tapestry of shared experiences that help make others feel seen, validated, and understood.

I have a handful of accounts I regularly look to, to stay informed on current food allergy issues. These include food allergy influencers who feel like friends I can turn to for understanding, even though our interactions are solely online. This digital camaraderie has fostered a sense of community I have never experienced before.

Social media has quickly become a powerful tool in spreading awareness. From quick tips on avoiding allergens to stories of resilience, helpful content circulates widely, amplifying our voices. These platforms give rise to a chorus demanding attention, where whispers of caution can no longer be ignored.

Building bridges of empathy and understanding across the landscape of those with disabilities, allergies, and dietary restrictions allows the public to step into our shoes, even if only briefly, to grasp the reality of living with a food allergy, which is crucial for fostering broader understanding. This newfound comprehension fosters empathy and compassion, making our challenges a collective concern and responsibility. Positive portrayals humanize our precautions—scrutinizing labels, navigating social gatherings—and highlight the courage it takes to navigate a world where a simple meal can become a life-threatening risk.

The implications of public awareness and understanding extend far beyond empathy alone. They impact public health and safety in profound ways. Improved awareness means restaurant staff can better accommodate dietary needs, schools can implement safer practices for allergic students, and emergency responders can swiftly recognize and respond to allergic reactions. Heightened awareness empowers communities to be vigilant and proactive, potentially saving lives in critical moments.

With 1 in 10 adults and 1 in 13 children navigating the complexities of food allergies, all falling in a different spot on the reactivity spectrum, the importance of meaningful and accurate portrayals cannot be overstated. Through the power of the media, we turn awareness into action, working toward a world where people with food allergies can feel acknowledged.

If you're looking for specific examples of positive and resonant food allergy portrayals in media, I have several resources to get you started:

- Food Allergy Canada's commercial "First Kiss": A heartfelt depiction that underscores the social challenges those with food allergies face. I felt seen by this, and knew I could share it with someone without a food allergy so they could better understand the experience.
- FARE's "Your Guide to Food Allergy" video: Offers

comprehensive practical advice and allergy representation. Additionally, FARE has a YouTube channel with a wealth of resources, including their 2023 campaign "It's Personal for Us" and back-to-school resource videos for managing food allergies in educational settings.

- End Allergies Together: "Could you eat?" The video brings awareness to the severity of food allergies, fosters empathy and understanding from those without allergies, and makes individuals feel less alone and validated. The video highlights their daily struggles, advocates for greater assistance, and encourages others to join the fight against food allergies.

- Andrea-Rachel Nt'l Commercial: Seeing the "Face your Risk" video taught me that every 6 minutes, life-threatening allergies send someone to the ER. As of 2024, though, the frequency of emergency room visits due to life-threatening allergic reactions has increased. According to Allergy & Asthma Network, currently an ER visit for food-induced anaphylaxis occurs approximately every 2-3 minutes in the United States. This marks a significant increase from earlier statistics, underscoring the growing prevalence and severity of food allergies and other anaphylactic reactions. You can check the sources End Allergies Together and Allergy & Asthma Network for more detailed information.

- Phoebe Campbell-Harris's short film, *A Matter of Minutes*: Partnering up with Natasha's Foundation (@natashasfoundation) and SlickFilms (@_slickfilms), this short film based around a kiss at a Paris nightclub that led to a medical emergency due to her food allergy shows a representation of a real-life situation.

- Everyday Allergen-Free: Amanda Orlando is the creator behind *Everyday Allergen-Free*. Through her writing, books, and social media presence, Amanda offers a thoughtful, honest, and deeply relatable look into life with food allergies. She's the author of multiple beautifully written books, which offer recipes, personal reflections, and practical tips for navigating allergies with confidence and creativity. Her website, everydayallergenfree.com, is full of resources, recipes, and writing that feel like a conversation with a trusted friend. Amanda's voice has helped shape a more inclusive and empowering allergy space, and I always appreciate her ability to blend vulnerability, advocacy, and everyday life in such a grounded, authentic way. She's Canadian and has expressed how Food Allergy Canada is an excellent resource she's relied on. Be sure to follow along with her non-profit, Free To Be Me Society.

- Allergies With Mia: Food Allergy Content Creator & Speaker (@allergieswithmia) on platforms like Instagram and TikTok. I've felt so much less alone after finding Mia's content on social media. I admire her empowering attitude, her approachable energy, and her gift for diving into niche, under-discussed allergy topics with clarity and care. She's always on the pulse of the latest trends, not afraid to take.a stance, and somehow still manages to make it all feel intimate—like you're texting with a friend who just gets it. And I'm lucky enough that we *do* text!

- InvisiblyAllergic.com: My own website was created to foster connection and understanding around the food allergy experience. Check out the topics on my blog and the resources section, which includes links to other helpful sites, ensuring you have access to a broad range of support and information.

Advocacy Efforts and Impact

Advocacy often feels overwhelming and like a big word, but there are many ways to advocate for a cause, and I wholeheartedly believe there is something everyone can do. Advocating could be talking to your non-allergic children, "How will you support your friend with allergies at school?" "What can we bring your friend with allergies for their birthday to make them feel special and non-food related?" "What do you do if your friend starts to have an allergic reaction?" Many people are surprised when I tell them that you're a food allergy ally just talking about allergies in the real world.

If you're a teacher, you become an ally by talking to your students about food allergies. Friends show allyship when they ask how to help accommodate someone's needs. Even asking restaurants about cross-contact practices or whether they use top allergens raises awareness and makes a difference.

Remarkably, advocacy efforts have profoundly transformed the landscape of food allergy awareness in recent years. Organizations like FAACT, AAFA, CFAAR, FARE, Allergy & Asthma Network, and others have been at the forefront, leading impactful campaigns and initiatives to increase understanding and support for those with food allergies. Their work ranges from spearheading national awareness campaigns and driving legislative change to developing vital educational resources—all in an effort to shape public policy and shift societal attitudes.

While FARE has historically played a significant role in these efforts, recent concerns within the community about leadership decisions and policy priorities have prompted many to reevaluate their support. The sudden loss of their internal advocacy team without communication to the community around it—many of whom had built strong relationships with advocates in the allergy community—has left a noticeable gap.

As always, it's important that we as individuals stay informed and critically engaged with our favorite non-profits, including those we've long trusted. Advocacy organizations evolve, and it's up to us to ensure the missions and policies they support continue to align with the needs and values of the communities they exist for and support.

Similarly, community-driven campaigns and social media

movements have empowered individuals to advocate for their rights and spotlight the food allergy community's challenges. These grassroots efforts amplify voices, educate the public, and drive systemic changes prioritizing the well-being of those with food allergies. By highlighting these advocacy efforts, I aim to showcase the transformative power of collective action in shaping public perceptions and policies related to food allergies and beyond.

Social media has revolutionized how we connect and share experiences, both in our communities and globally. I believe this digital community has been incredible in shaping how I view my food allergy experience. Before social media, I felt like I was stranded on an island. Discovering accounts like Amanda Orlando's *Everyday Allergen-Free*, which shares allergy-aware recipe ideas and relatable personal insights, and Allergies With Mia, where I could see someone else living a day-to-day life similar to mine, has made me feel less alone and more empowered.

Social media is a powerful tool for advocacy and education, with individuals like Amanda and Mia, and organizations such as FAACT and Food Allergy Canada leading the way. They use these platforms to share personal stories, debunk myths, and advocate for inclusive policies, empowering the food allergy community and fostering broader societal change, promoting understanding and accessibility for all.

However, social media isn't inclusive of all disabilities and isn't the only way to advocate.

Taking action in your community, through local in-person efforts or other ways, can be equally effective and fulfilling. While my experience with social media has connected me to others globally and provided valuable resources, there are many ways to find support and advocate for change. The most important thing is to take action in whatever way feels meaningful and authentic to you, and to speak up in a manner that feels comfortable if you encounter friction from negative portrayals, offensive media, or dangerous misinformation.

Closing Thoughts & Additional Context

- Recent Incidents: Controversies like the 2024 Super Bowl commercial, the movies *The Roses* and *Freakier Friday,* and insensitive public remarks underscore the ongoing challenges in combating misinformation and stigma surrounding food allergies.

- Positive Portrayals: Initiatives by organizations like Food Allergy Canada and FARE, including heartfelt commercials and educational videos, humanize the experiences of those with food allergies, fostering empathy and understanding.

- Impact on Public Health: Accurate media representations about food allergies and allergic reactions, such as anaphylaxis, empower communities to implement safer practices in restaurants, schools, and emergency settings, thereby enhancing safety for those with food allergies. Misinformation in the media can cause confusion and undermine efforts to provide necessary accommodations.

- Role of Social Media: Platforms like Instagram and YouTube enable food allergy influencers to provide crucial resources and community for individuals managing food allergies. That's been my aim with my own social media accounts, @invisiblyallergic, to create a place someone can come to when they're feeling misunderstood, lonely, or struggling to get their food allergies under control. While specific platforms may change over time, the trend of raising awareness and building community spans across all social media, including Substack and other emerging spaces.

- Advocacy and Education: By advocating for responsible media representation and leveraging social platforms for education and advocacy, we can drive meaningful change for the global food allergy community. For those creating media involving food allergy depictions, I offer free consulting services on my website that provide guidance to ensure accurate and respectful portrayals.

- A Life Cut Short: Órla Baxendale: The tragic death of Órla Baxendale in New York City in January 2024 highlights the importance of accurate labeling. Órla, a 25-year-old dancer, died after experiencing anaphylactic shock after eating a mislabeled cookie that contained peanuts but did not have peanuts listed in the ingredients panel. She was from the EU, where there are safer, more comprehensive food labeling laws that she was likely used to being able to rely on. Food allergy non-profits have often explained to me that the US is "currently decades behind the EU in terms of labeling law requirements."

11

THE INTERSECTION OF MENTAL HEALTH AND FOOD ALLERGIES

Mental Health through a Food Allergy Lens

Throughout this book, I've aimed to shed light on the profound impact of food allergies on mental health. In Chapter 2, I touched on the troubling issue of food allergy bullying, a persistent problem that affects individuals regardless of age or life stage. In this chapter, I further explore the topic of bullying to offer strategies specific to food allergies.

I'm purposefully discussing mental health in broad strokes, sharing insights from the resources I've picked up in the community, not as a medical professional. Since it's not my skill set to discuss mental health as a professional, I aim not to provide super specific, targeted advice. Instead, I strive to offer a clear jumping point for conversations with your licensed therapist or mental health professional, as neither therapy nor managing food allergies is one-size-fits-all.

I've observed that in today's culture, we've grown more comfortable discussing the "lighter" aspects of mental health, such as self-care, but heavier topics like mental illness—particularly suicide and other stigmatized conditions—still feel taboo. I hope for a more open and honest future where conversations happen around all aspects of mental health and mental illness, especially the heavy ones, as avoiding these discussions does a disservice to those struggling silently.

I hope one day the general public without allergies will have more of an understanding of the intricate relationship between food allergies and mental health, to foster a supportive and inclusive environment long-term for the food allergy community and their impacted social circles. I believe by improving food and non-food labeling practices for allergen transparency, increasing requirements of all accommodations, and promoting accurate allergy media representation, much of the anxiety and stress experienced by those with food allergies could be alleviated.

The truth is, that living with food allergies profoundly impacts mental health in several ways, which vary from person to person. Some common examples are feelings of sorrow, exclusion, anxiety, fear, and stress. This chapter explores some aspects of the psychological toll of navigating a world that frequently lacks even the most foundational accommodations and understanding of the life-threatening food allergy experience. Furthermore, I want to focus on how witnessing others with food allergies not being accommodated, or experiencing the lack of inclusion ourselves, can be deeply traumatic. Unfortunately, the absence of proper labeling across all products, coupled with insufficient healthcare and social services—including mental health care—adds to this trauma.

I understand these struggles intimately; and writing this book has been both a healing process and a challenge, as delving deeply into these issues can be extremely bleak. If you have or manage a food allergy, I hope this chapter validates your feelings of potential ostracism, as well as any struggles. Using our voices to keep food allergy hurdles as topics of conversation, will help push for better labeling practices, increased accommodations, more robust mental health support, and who even knows what else. There is power in our testimonies and collective advocacy, and together, we can drive meaningful change.

Despite all the hurdles, I remain filled with hope and empowerment. I am the type of person who sees how cruel and unfair our world can be in individual ways and global ways—and I do dwell on it—but I also can't help but be amazed at the miraculousness that we're even here at all in the first place.

Being treated as the odd one out, fearing reactions, enduring mockery, and struggling with a lack of empathy or resistance to accommodations—these are just some of the ways life with food allergies can be emotionally taxing. These circumstances and events could be explored endlessly: fear of the auto-injector, hesitation around when to use or not use epinephrine, and the physical and mental recovery after anaphylaxis.

The cycle of food allergy stress extends far beyond what many may imagine, which is usually the physical risks of an allergic reaction. It's a struggle for safety, inclusion, and acceptance in daily life—something I hope others without allergies can recognize and validate for the food allergy community.

As you've likely noticed, a main focus of mine related to food allergy mental health is the inadequate labeling of both food and non-food items in the US, including products one might assume are already labeled for top allergens, such as medications, skin and beauty products, and alcoholic beverages. This lack of transparency, discussed in depth in Chapters 7–9, poses serious risks, making it incredibly difficult for consumers to make informed decisions to help mitigate life-threatening allergic reactions. The uncertainty caused by the lack of critical allergen information takes a significant mental toll on individuals and their families. Plus, frequent news reports of anaphylactic-related deaths—many of which could have been prevented—only add to the emotional overwhelm felt within the community.

This is further compounded in the US by the significant financial strain of life-saving medications, such as epinephrine. With prices reaching upward of $600 per 2-pack, even with insurance, and exceeding $1,000+ per 2-pack without, the burden only grows. This doesn't account for the need to replace them annually due to expiration, or potentially multiple times over, if used. I recently spoke to a family who had gone through 10+ injectors in three months while they struggled to pinpoint their daughter's newly developed allergies, which fell outside of the top 9.

This chapter provides a magnifying lens of the intricate relationship between food allergies and the mental health challenges and mental illnesses that can arise from them, like anxiety disorders, depression, or post-traumatic stress disorder (PTSD). As these challenges become more apparent, so does the need for comprehensive support and advocacy. By pointing out these interconnected issues, I hope to empower those living with food allergies and mobilize their networks—families, friends, caregivers, and professionals—who can all help to advocate for meaningful change towards a more inclusive society that recognizes the allergy reactivity spectrum and the holistic impact of living with food allergies.

The Psychological Impact

Food allergy living feels like a delicate tightrope between gratitude and hopelessness, heightened by the ever-present threat of unexpected loss of life. This balancing act can show up in different ways, from feeling impatient with certain life events and goals to pushing ourselves to live life fully every day—even when we're too tired and need to rest. I know I struggle with envy, jealousy, and a tendency to compare myself to others in an unhelpful way. Some days merely surviving can be a challenge—not only in terms of what I eat, but also in avoiding cross-contact or accidental exposure in various public and private environments. Acknowledging this weight helps me to manage it and try to practice self-love and gratitude in response. It also keeps my inner critic in check.

Just as the greater disability community advocates for open discussions about disabilities without stigmatizing the term and not treating it as a "bad word," I believe we should approach conversations about food allergies candidly in the same spirit. I've been told on social media by others that this transparent approach is fearmongering, but I think addressing the topic of death is important for so many reasons.

I'm not saying you need to discuss this with children or teens before it's an appropriate age or bring it up at times when it would make someone anxious, but talking about death is a part of living life with an IgE-mediated food allergy. Simply put, ignoring this aspect when someone has a life-threatening allergy hinders others' accurate understanding of this complex condition. In the past, I've tried to brush off this intense part of myself, which did nothing but manifest it as shame and guilt while trying to pretend it wasn't a part of me.

Ultimately, my therapist helped me realize that I was hiding this somber part of myself for the sake of others, and it had me constantly putting myself second. The truth is, I face a real risk of easily dying. It's uncomfortable to bring up when it's not talked about at all, but instead of pushing it down, I can share how it is my reality and explain how to use my epinephrine and signs of anaphylaxis. This openness allows others to connect with me on a deeper level, and since vulnerability is a core value I hold, it's led to such deep friendships in a way I've only ever dreamed of experiencing.

My perspective is undoubtedly shaped by living with an anaphylactic food allergy since childhood, and I recognize that this experience may not resonate with everyone across the reactivity spectrum, but it is the reality for many. I'm sharing this because I found that openly acknowledging this weight of death, rather than hiding it, helped me lighten it.

Over the years, I've noticed a crossover between people with celiac disease and those with food allergies, and I've learned a great deal from the online celiac community. I've especially learned from social media influencers who raise awareness about the severity of their condition, which is often dismissed as merely causing "a tummy ache." For many with celiac, gluten contamination can lead to debilitating symptoms such as joint pain, vomiting, dizziness, and migraines, which can persist for days. This is why I make it an effort to validate everyone's experiences, regardless of whether or not they face anaphylactic reactions. There's no hierarchy of importance when it comes to bodily conditions, each experience is valid and deserves respect.

Each individual's struggle carries its weight, and recognizing the seriousness of these chronic conditions is essential, as they profoundly impact lives and quality of life in ways that may not be immediately visible. It's easy to dismiss someone else's challenges if they don't align exactly with our own experiences, especially if they conflict with them. However, this mindset overlooks the complexity of suffering.

True empathy requires us to look beyond our own experiences and recognize that everyone faces unique challenges. I often grapple with this, sometimes becoming too insular within my peanut allergy perspective. I don't always embody the compassion I aim to show, and I continue to work on expanding my understanding beyond my bubble. I truly believe that although we may not fully understand another person's struggles, we can all acknowledge our shared humanity. By embracing this perspective, we can foster an environment of understanding that uplifts us all, regardless of the nature or severity of their condition. Our shared experiences can unite us instead of dividing us, reminding us that while our journeys differ, the need for validation and compassion remains a universal necessity we all deserve. And I don't just mean in the US, but across the globe.

Through my years of therapy with a couple different therapists, I have come to recognize the vital role of self-compassion in my life. I've found significant value in therapeutic techniques, such as Eye Movement Desensitization and Reprocessing (EMDR) and Internal Family Systems (IFS) therapy, especially at this stage of my likely lifelong journey with anxiety. I share these approaches here as potential avenues for others to explore with a qualified mental health professional.

It's important to remember that there are many modality options when addressing the intersection of food allergies and mental health and mental illness—what works for one person may not work for another, and it may take time to find the most suitable therapeutic approach. If you haven't yet found one that fits, I encourage you to keep exploring different forms of therapy, and if you have, hooray! Sticking with various therapeutic approaches has helped me discover what resonates most deeply with me, leading to a transformative experience where I feel truly seen.

Self-Advocacy

Those managing food allergies face a continuous backward and forward between self-advocacy and mental health. On one hand, advocating for oneself is essential to ensure safety and communicate needs to others that wouldn't otherwise be known. This requires a proactive approach, where individuals must explain their dietary restrictions and educate those around them about the seriousness of their condition. However, this self-advocacy can be laborious and often does not come naturally, especially when facing resistance or lack of understanding from others.

On the other hand, it's also important to recognize and accept that not everyone may be willing or able to accommodate us. Striking a balance between advocating for oneself and managing the expectations of others is crucial for maintaining mental health amidst food allergies.

One primary effect is chronic anxiety and stress arising from the relentless vigilance required to avoid allergens. Individuals with food allergies remain perpetually alert, always checking ingredients and assessing potentially hazardous environments. This constant scrutiny offers no breaks, even in one's own home, as outside influences can bring a certain level of contamination inside. If it's not coming into the house on our clothes, it's coming in on our purses, shopping bags, shoes, and more. It's inevitable in most cases, unless we immediately put all our clothes in the wash and wipe everything down with a wet wipe, which I'm not doing.

This aspect of food allergy life can be mentally depleting. In my experience, as well as what I've observed in others, this heightened state of awareness leads to quicker fatigue and amplifies other sources of stress and anxiety. For example, I find that when I travel, I invest significantly more mental energy into managing my day-to-day compared to my routine life at home. As a result, it often takes me several days to mentally recover afterward—I need a mini "vacation" from my "vacation."

Feeling Like a Burden

Social challenges can exacerbate the psychological impact of living with food allergies. Many with allergies, as well as their families, often feel isolated or excluded due to their dietary restrictions. To protect themselves, they might choose to avoid social gatherings or events they genuinely wish to attend. While such avoidance can be necessary for safety, it can, on top of that, lead to feelings of loneliness and a sense of missing out on meaningful interactions.

This pattern of exclusion can greatly diminish a person's sense of connection with others and intensify feelings of being left out, especially when it occurs repeatedly rather than as a one-time occurrence. As we now know from recent data collected around connection, the *American Journal of Public Health* from 2023 found that being a part of a supportive community can activate your body's repair genes, reduce inflammation, and even extend your lifespan. This field known as sociogenomics, which studies how social factors affect the genome, has found that a sense of connection can improve mental health and decision-making skills. To learn more, check out the latest in the *American Journal of Sociogenomics.*

When discussing the mental hurdles related to food allergies, the effects on self-worth and identity come to the forefront of my mind. This is a frequent topic discussed in my therapy sessions, as I navigate my lifelong peanut allergy, over 35 years in. Many individuals with food allergies grapple with deep internal conflicts, including anxiety, alienation, and a diminished sense of self. These struggles are often tied to experiences of exclusion and the perception of being a burden to others, which can profoundly shape one's identity and overall well-being.

I sometimes struggle with self-advocacy around prioritizing my food allergy needs and will default to people-pleasing. I worry about appearing entitled or demanding, which can make it difficult for me to request the accommodations I want. In the past, I've had this problem advocating for myself in the workplace and college settings, which I feel much more confident in now, but in other areas of my personal life, the challenge still remains.

I feel much more comfortable advocating for others' needs rather than my own, so practicing advocating for myself as if I were advocating for a friend is one tactic I use. Plus, in many situations, I've come to understand that many people may genuinely want to accommodate me, but simply don't know how, and need to know my accommodation preferences, but don't know how to ask. I can relate to this hesitation, as I often choose not to say anything for the same reasons.

Sometimes I feel silly and over-reactive for removing myself from a situation, only to find out there were no peanuts present after all. For instance, the sound of a wrapper made me think someone was eating a peanut butter candy bar or a peanut-like smell that turned out to be something else entirely.

During a podcast interview I did on *Behind The Allergy,* I brought this up, and the host shared something that reassured me. She shared that her inner narrative in these potentially hyper-sensitive moments is more like, "So what if I removed myself from a situation and it turns out I didn't need to? So what if others think I overreacted?" Essentially, she doesn't regret putting her needs first and removing herself in those moments. This perspective was comforting. It reminded me that prioritizing my well-being and advocating for my needs is nothing to feel guilty about.

After all, sometimes the sound really is a peanut wrapper, and the smell really is peanuts—so it makes sense to be cautious. Feeling guilty about overreacting about my allergy is a recurring struggle. I can be told repeatedly I have nothing to feel guilty about, yet I do wrestle with those feelings and the notion that I'm a burden. Even though I know deep down I'd do the same for others and not see them as a burden, I still grapple with the perception that I'm an inconvenience and that it may just be easier for me to not even try to be accommodated.

I think this stems from challenging the "norm," disrupting what society has trained us to come to expect, so it feels different, and that difference can feel stressful compared to what life might be like without my cross-contact and airborne peanut allergy. Now that I know it may seem like "overreacting" to the general public, in fact my reaction is an appropriate response to my food allergy. Many in the space, such as those who don't deal with it all the time or parents who can take a vacation from managing their kids' allergies and then post about eating their kids' allergens on the trips, don't have the same constant responsibility. No shade, but it's important to acknowledge that there *is* a difference. That doesn't mean I'm not worth the effort.

At a recent food allergy conference, I asked a question to a food allergy expert in the space who attends many conferences as a coveted speaker each year. I wondered if airborne aspects of food allergies, as well as any reactions to food that are outside of traditional ingesting of allergens, is something she hears being talked about. Cross-contact to me is such a huge part of managing my allergy and avoiding reactions, so I was curious. She said it was not a topic she heard mentioned frequently, if at all. I found this interesting and likely see it as something that will continue being discussed more as the allergic field continues to better understand the allergic person's experience.

I may go for weeks or even months feeling secure in my self-worth, but that confidence can quickly crumble when someone refuses to accommodate my needs—especially on days when my mental state is already fragile. This can send me spiraling back into food allergy anxiety. Something as simple as planning a vacation requires a great deal of effort because of my allergy, and it impacts not just me but my partner, too. Our options for flights, hotels, and destinations are dependent on how we may best be able to avoid my allergen and align with financial implications. We select airlines and hotels based on that instead of our ideal price point. What could be a carefree trip instead turns into careful, detailed planning, with spontaneity taking a backseat to ensure my safety. But does my partner mind? Not at all. After a decade together, he knows what to expect—this is just how we travel, whether visiting family or taking a vacation.

Yes, it takes extra planning and may not look like the usual experiences around eating, but it's okay. In life, I try to focus on the experiences and small wins rather than the meals. Sometimes a day or trip is food-focused, which can be fun, but it doesn't *have to be*. I remind myself of this, especially in unfamiliar environments when I'm out of my comfort zone. There's almost always a peanut-free chain restaurant, convenience store, or grocery store with options. I do tend to over-plan and seek out safe restaurants when I travel, even for a quick trip, even when it's not always necessary. So, I'm making a mental note to remind myself that it's okay to let go of that pressure sometimes and just enjoy the moment and eat the food we've brought from a store. I'm mentally filing that tiny piece of self-guidance away for later.

In exploring my own identity as a person with a life-threatening food allergy, I often wonder how much my passion for social advocacy has been shaped by that experience. Advocacy and empathy has been an integral part of myself since childhood. From organizing a PETA protest in my neighborhood to oppose animal cruelty toward the chickens used by Kentucky Fried Chicken, to going on a family vacation with a friend's family to Florida and coming back deeply inspired to help injured manatees affected by boaters. I eagerly contributed my allowances to help rehabilitate a manatee named Rosie, who was assigned to me for many years. These early experiences ignited a spark within me, inspiring a commitment to stand up for a wide range of social justice causes ever since.

I find purpose and fulfillment in volunteering and helping look out for others' long-term well-being, yet it often carries a level of sadness that lingers and keeps me up at night. Witnessing the pain and suffering associated with various causes does lead to my own bouts with depression, but this is something I'm used to, as it mirrors the duality of my peanut allergy. While I grapple with managing what to do with these heavy emotions, I simultaneously feel a sense of hope, resilience, and gratitude.

Over the years, I've often questioned whether I'm a "highly sensitive person," as a result of my lifelong anaphylactic food allergy. I also ponder the relationship between my generalized anxiety and my allergy: *Am I inherently an anxious person, or is my anxiety a byproduct of managing a serious, life-threatening condition? Would I worry this much if I hadn't grown up with such a significant allergy?* These questions have occupied my thoughts repeatedly, and while I may never find definitive answers, I've come to accept that uncertainty is part of many people's lives and my own story.

Yet, nothing good has ever come to me from stewing in a negative mindset for too long. I can acknowledge the challenges and allow myself a small but impressive pity party, but make sure to avoid sitting in those feelings for too long, as they can escalate into an anxious-depressive state. A local artist in my community once shared a thought that resonated deeply with me: "No matter how bad something is, try to find some happiness and not let yourself have a bad 24 hours." My goal is to acknowledge these emotions while staying curious and present. I often remind myself that just because I have a thought about something, this doesn't mean it's factual.

Cultivating gratitude in small moments throughout my day has been a helpful way to balance my overall stress. And I've learned that each challenge presents an opportunity for growth and resilience, and it's okay to feel sad and grieve sometimes. Moreover, I recognize that everyone has their struggles and that perfection is an illusion, which aids me in managing the extra planning and energy my food allergy demands.

Managing a food allergy—or multiple allergies or additional conditions—while striving to maintain a positive self-image can feel like a constant seesaw, with extreme ups and downs. Embracing self-compassion and celebrating small victories keeps me grounded, reminding me that I am more than my allergy. This mindset allows me to confront deeper issues, such as the connection between food allergies and the heightened risk of developing eating disorders that many individuals face in their quest for safety and control.

I see how easily eating disorders and food allergies intertwine, twist, and knot in complex, tangled ways. Research indicates that individuals with food allergies may be at a higher risk of developing disordered eating patterns. This overlap often stems from the restrictive nature of managing allergies, which can inadvertently increase fixation on food, body weight, and body image. The continued use of the widely applied term BMI (body mass index), despite being challenged by many in the medical community for being considered outdated and inaccurate, exacerbates this issue.

For one, BMI fails to distinguish between muscle and fat or indicate fat distribution in the body, which significantly limits its accuracy in assessing health risks. In June 2023, The American

Medical Association (AMA) recognized that BMI alone is an insufficient measure of health and is advocating for a change in clinical practice. In response, the AMA adopted a new policy acknowledging the issues with using BMI as a measurement, citing its historical harm and use for racist exclusion. Healthcare professionals are more regularly encouraged to use BMI only in conjunction with other measures such as waist circumference, blood pressure, and cholesterol levels for a more comprehensive health evaluation.

A systematic review published in 2023 in *The Journal of Allergy & Clinical Immunology: In Practice* investigated the prevalence of eating disorders among individuals with food allergies. The review encompassed 4,161 adult and pediatric participants with food allergies. The findings suggest that eating disorders such as avoidant/restrictive food intake disorder (ARFID), anorexia nervosa, and bulimia nervosa may be common among children and adults with food allergies.

While the exact prevalence remains unclear due to variations in study methods, the review highlights that disordered eating behaviors are something to watch among people with food allergies. The study found that food allergy has been associated with a range of these behaviors, including excessively limited diets, feeding aversions, and limited psychosocial functioning around food and meals.

Separately, other eating-related conditions are sometimes discussed in the allergy space. Binge eating disorder is DSM-5 recognized, while orthorexia nervosa is not yet an official DSM-5 diagnosis. Fear-based food conditions also exist, including cibophobia (fear of food), phagophobia (fear of swallowing), and food neophobia (fear of trying new foods). These conditions are not formally recognized as disorders in the DSM-5 as of the date of this book's publishing, but can still significantly affect eating behaviors and quality of life.

A prior study published in the 2015 *Journal of Allergy and Clinical Immunology* found that up to 22% of adolescents with food allergies exhibited symptoms indicative of feeding and eating challenges, such as avoiding food altogether or adopting extreme dietary restrictions. You can see this is a somewhat studied topic, but still isn't well understood. This is just something we're realizing needs to be watched out for in the allergy community.

I can see how there's a psychological strain in constantly navigating food choices, which tends to lift the veil on feelings of insecurity and further complicates one's relationship with food. While managing food allergies is essential for safety, it can sometimes evolve into an unhealthy preoccupation that detracts from overall well-being.

If someone reading this is experiencing these symptoms, seeking guidance from licensed professionals—such as a registered dietitian or therapist—can be an excellent step. These experts provide holistic support and tailored advice to navigate both the practicalities of allergy management and the emotional landscape surrounding food. I've found that getting referrals from friends, family, or trusted colleagues helps me find someone I can trust. Engaging with professionals about my food allergy struggles has led to healthier coping strategies, promoted a more balanced perspective on food, and ultimately fostered a more positive relationship with myself.

Admittedly, as I've entered my mid 30s, I've become more self-conscious about my body image and occasionally struggle with negative thoughts about my appearance, as I struggle to fit into my usual clothes—many of which come with the natural territory of aging. While I know these feelings are completely normal, I still feel frustrated by the changes in my body that I'm not quite used to. In the pursuit to be totally transparent, I say this because I do have a habit of emotional eating, which I try to keep an eye on.

Sometimes I will bulk buy a safe food product that is hard

to find and then overindulge in it, eating my feelings when I'm stressed and not even when I'm feeling hungry. This especially happens if it's something like an ice cream sandwich or a super yummy dessert.

Alongside my emotional eating habits, I sometimes notice a scarcity complex within myself. I strive to practice generosity and avoid hoarding food, but this tendency can flare up, especially when I feel frustrated about not finding safe food brands and products. When I do discover something safe, I may feel compelled to stock up on it—even if it's unhealthy or unnecessary, like buying multiple boxes of different varieties of safe ice cream cones that are readily available year-round at my local grocery store. I have to watch my habits and patterns, so I don't go overboard.

Part of this urge comes from wanting to reinforce the need to the store in continuing to carry those items, but it can lead to upset stomachs or wasted food, resulting in guilt. This cycle is something I've discussed in both therapy and with a dietitian. My food allergy often makes me possessive about food, too. If I make something safe, or someone makes me something safe, I may not want to share it.

I hope that by sharing my vulnerable internal struggles here, I can help normalize having open conversations around these types of topics. It's important to note that not every individual with food allergies, or their families, will have the same experiences I've described here. By fostering a better understanding of the psychological impact of food allergies among both medical and psychological professionals, as well as society at large, we can acknowledge the multifaceted challenges faced by those living with these conditions daily. Moreover, we can emphasize the importance of proactively addressing mental health needs with the seriousness and validity they deserve.

If you're new to navigating food allergies, whether it's one or many, eating may feel bland at first and less enjoyable while your taste buds adjust and you discover new recipes that work for you. But I promise, it does get better. With time, creativity, and support, your meals will become joyful and even craveworthy again.

Coping Strategies: Daily Life with Food Allergies

Each encounter with potential allergens can evoke a profound sense of vulnerability and panic over a possible danger. Something I've found that is less frequently discussed in the food allergy space is how this persistent state of alertness in those managing allergies can mirror the hyper-awareness often experienced by trauma survivors and individuals living with post-traumatic stress disorder (PTSD). A 2020 National Library of Medicine article found that people with severe food allergies often develop heightened vigilance to manage physical and social risks associated with allergic reactions. This vigilance stems from embodied memories of past reactions and an imagination of potential dangers.

Trauma can manifest in various ways, including hypervigilance, flashbacks, avoidance behaviors, difficulty concentrating, and a heightened startle response. While there is research on phobias of anaphylaxis, studies specifically addressing trauma caused by food allergies remain scarce. This gap leaves many of us navigating the psychological toll of living with food allergies without a clear understanding of how it aligns with broader trauma responses.

We know that experiencing or witnessing anaphylaxis can be traumatic, leading to PTSD symptoms such as flashbacks, avoidance behaviors, and hyperarousal. These symptoms include being constantly on edge, easily startled, and excessively scanning the environment for threats—behaviors that align closely with those managing severe food allergies.

Both PTSD and the management of life-threatening food allergies involve significant psychological stress. For example, individuals with PTSD exhibit hyperarousal symptoms like irritability, insomnia, and difficulty concentrating, which are also common in people managing severe allergies due to their constant need to avoid triggers and ensure safety.

This mental and emotional alertness is not only fatiguing but also significantly impacts one's overall well-being, much like any other trauma-related trigger. In exploring this connection out of my own curiosity, I found profound insights in Bessel van der Kolk's book, *The Body Keeps the Score*.

His examination of the intricate interplay between trauma and the body reveals how traumatic experiences can become deeply embedded in both our minds and our physiology. Van der Kolk's insights into how trauma alters brain function and shapes emotional responses resonated deeply with me, concerning the daily challenges I face with my peanut allergy. Therefore, this next part of the chapter focuses on practical coping strategies and tools, to encourage a sense of safety and resilience in a world filled with tangible and legitimate potential triggers.

I enjoyed reading van der Kolk's holistic approach to healing—encompassing psychological therapies like CBT, EMDR, and somatic treatments—which explained how these can provide a valuable framework for understanding and managing the mental health impacts of various chronic health conditions.

Since first reading *The Body Keeps the Score*, I've learned more about concerns that have been raised regarding van der Kolk himself. He was ultimately dismissed from the Trauma Center he founded following allegations of bullying and demeaning staff, had patient complaints, and questions around his scientific integrity, to the point where he's no longer affiliated with Harvard. I still think his book offers a useful framework for understanding trauma and healing, but I recommend it with the caveat that there are many other excellent mental health books available as well. Personally, I like to browse Libby, the free library app, to explore what resonates with my own needs and interests, from voices outside of the predominately white male lens, since mental health writing spans such a wide spectrum of approaches and voices.

Through reading the 2018 book *The Deepest Well* by Dr. Nadine Burke Harris, MD, I learned that childhood adversity "can have life-long effects. Twenty years of medical research has shown it changes us in ways that impact our bodies for decades: it can tip a child's developmental trajectory, affect physiology, trigger chronic inflammation and hormonal changes that last a lifetime, alter the way DNA is read and how cells replicate."

I highly recommend this book to anyone—you may know Dr. Burke Harris from her popular TED talk on Adverse Childhood Experiences (ACEs). Her expertise lies in quantifying adversity so we can understand our risk levels accordingly, and the insights I gained about ACEs blew me away. For example, a person with an ACE score of 2 or more has twice the odds of hospitalization for autoimmune disease compared with someone with a score of 0.

Most people don't think about conditions as being caused by anything other than bad luck, and as she explains, it's harder to connect diseases like Graves disease or Multiple sclerosis (MS) to trauma until we understand how it impacts the body. She writes, "it is counter to the story they may already have in their heads. Those with high ACEs were shown to be at higher risk of depression, anxiety, asthma, autoimmune disease, food allergies, cardiac disease, fibromyalgia, stomach ulcers, and the list goes on." She wrote her book for "all the caretakers in the world to give the children in their care the best shot despite life's difficulties," and I admired reading about her story and career.

Another critical aspect of living with a food allergy—or multiple allergies—that I've only slightly scratched the surface of before is the importance of maintaining a balanced diet. With the growing emphasis on healthy, clean eating, we're becoming increasingly aware of its profound impact on our mindset and gut health, which, in turn, affects our brain function, mood, and immune system. In the US, in September, we celebrate "Food is Medicine Day," underscoring the necessity of regular access to nutritious foods for overall well-being.

For those newly diagnosed with a food allergy, as well as families experienced in managing multiple allergies, crafting a healthy diet requires meticulous attention, particularly when navigating ingredient substitutions and exclusions.

Often if you have a food allergy, an oral food challenge, known as an OFC, is done at an allergist's office to confirm it. However, not always, as it depends on the patient's reaction history and interest in doing a challenge, upon other variables. Several recent studies have examined the impact of oral food challenges (OFCs) on the quality of life of individuals with food allergies.

Many found improved quality of life after doing an OFC, even if they react and use epinephrine, since they have answers and know what to expect with management. OFCs also allow participants to see how quickly symptoms subside after using an epi. However, OFCs can still be traumatizing for some. For example, an OFC might ease a parent's anxiety, while causing distress to the child who experienced the reaction, or vice versa.

I recently listened to a podcast interview with Dr. Ruchi Gupta on *Don't Feed the Fear*, where she shared how she uses a grapefruit to role-play administering expired epinephrine with her daughter's friends. I love this idea! It's a simple, hands-on way to build confidence and make emergency preparedness feel less intimidating. I plan to do the same with my own friends and family.

Dr. Gupta also talked about her family's own food allergy experiences, which reassured me. Hearing her stories normalized many of the challenges I face and helped soften my own guilt and self-critical thoughts. She highlighted some unexpected positives from a study on managing food allergies, such as healthier eating habits, increased empathy, and stronger advocacy skills.

There are so many things I genuinely appreciate and admire about Dr. Ruchi Gupta. She recognized early on that, as a society, we didn't fully understand the burden of food allergies—so she set out to fill that gap through research and advocacy even before her life was impacted by food allergies. Her work became even more personal when her own daughter had an allergic reaction to exposure to her brother's peanut butter and jelly sandwich. From that moment on, Dr. Gupta became a food allergy parent herself, deepening her commitment to the cause both professionally and personally. What I especially love about her approach is how she emphasizes improving quality of life now, in the day-to-day, as we await a cure or more preventive strategies. Her perspective that "we're doing the best we can with what we know" is so grounding and compassionate.

One of Dr. Gupta's studies on adults with food allergies found that nearly 50% developed at least one of their allergies as an adult. This challenges the common belief that food allergies are only a childhood issue. Researchers are exploring what might "turn on" these allergies in adulthood—some possible factors include hormonal shifts (during puberty, pregnancy, or menopause), significant illnesses that affect the immune system (like viral or bacterial infections), or even environmental changes such as moving to a new location. The microbiome is also being closely studied as a potential contributor to these changes. Some people lose food allergies after pregnancy, while others gain them—it's a complex and fascinating area of research, and I know I'll continue to follow Dr. Gupta's work closely as it evolves each year.

On a related note, Dr. Gupta's daughter currently attends a university with a nut-free cafeteria, and more schools are adopting similar policies, including Duke and Northwestern. For anyone interested, Spokin publishes an annual college guide with up-to-date information on allergy-friendly campuses. Food-allergic hardships aren't "worse" at any age, but they change with environment and independence. College brings new freedom, so resources that help navigate allergies safely and build self-advocacy are especially valuable.

A 2018 PubMed systematic review found that OFCs are associated with improved food allergy-specific health-related quality of life (HRQL) and reduced parental burden of food allergy. The review specifically noted that parent-reported HRQL improved significantly after an OFC, regardless of the outcome, in children with suspected food allergies. Overwhelmingly, the research taken so far indicates that for many, the benefits of having clear answers and management strategies outweigh the temporary stress of the procedure.

I know several individuals who manage 30+ food allergies, underscoring the urgent need for more formal, studied discussions on this topic. The nutritional balance of their diets can be significantly compromised, profoundly impacting their overall health and quality of life. This challenge is further complicated by the fact that many nutritionists, dietitians, allergists, and even the broader medical community often lack a comprehensive understanding of how cross-contact operates within our food system and lack knowledge of the proven types of strategies individuals in the food allergy community use to avoid it.

This knowledge gap is a key reason I wrote this book. It's not sufficient to simply check ingredients and nutrition labels; individuals with food allergies often also need to ask about allergens in the facilities where products are made. Since this information isn't required to be disclosed, what seems like a simple request becomes a bigger challenge than it should be—a topic I explored in depth in Chapters 6 and 7.

While there are resources available on maintaining a balanced diet with food allergies, such as PubMed, there is a need for more in-depth research and formal discussions around it. Especially for those managing multiple severe allergies, there needs to be more advanced care in this area.

Because this lack of ingredient transparency extends beyond food to prescriptions and non-food products like skincare, while we want to rely on pharmacists and the medical field to recommend safe options, they aren't trained to recognize allergens, and the laws aren't in place to help them understand the facilities and ingredients in these non-food products. This sense of distrust is valid, and it creates a tricky situation where, as the patient, I've usually felt more knowledgeable about certain allergy-related issues than my doctors or pharmacist. It's not a good feeling to have to be your own advocate in this way, and it's due to allergies being an understudied field and an unregulated topic.

Then there's the emotional impact of food allergies, particularly when linked to traumatic experiences, which cannot be overlooked. Experiencing an allergic reaction or even witnessing a distressing piece of food allergy social media news about a reaction, can evoke complex emotional responses, triggering vivid memories. I've learned that the individual may not just merely recall an experience but feel in their sympathetic nervous system as though they are reliving it—re-traumatizing them in the process. Science shows that traumatic memories tend to linger longer in our minds compared to positive ones, another thing I learned from the excellent book, *Uniquely Human*, about Autism.

A clinical trial in London is currently exploring the link between food allergies and children's mental health and cognition. The researchers hypothesize that allergic reactions may cause a post-traumatic stress disorder-like syndrome in children, potentially affecting hippocampal neurogenesis, a process linked to memory and mood regulation. The aftermath of an anaphylactic reaction can lead to prolonged hypervigilance, where people are afraid to eat anything offered by others, including parents, which can last for years.

These innermost negative memories can provoke panic or

heightened anxiety around food and eating, leading to emotional responses that may seem disproportionate or confusing to others without allergies. What may be labeled as "overdramatic" from the outside is often an unseen, deep-seated response to the ongoing trauma that food allergies can inflict.

Much like the expression, "the straw that broke the camel's back," the sympathetic nervous system's fight-or-flight response builds up internally, like a volcano under pressure. It can erupt as an outward expression of accumulated stress—at any moment. What can appear sudden, unexpected, and confusing to others is often the result of an allergic individual managing their stress and anxiety for a long time until it eventually becomes overwhelming.

I recall a comment someone made during a particularly challenging month of managing my allergies. We were traveling in a remote area with limited access to safe foods, and the food allergy stress was crushing me. I felt frustrated by the lack of options, isolated from those who could dine out freely, and unable to grab pre-made meals like everyone else was doing. It wasn't their fault, but I found myself internalizing these feelings, jealous and frustrated over my allergy limitations.

In the midst of this, I kept my emotions bottled up until someone casually said, "We just drove past a bakery. Why don't you call them? It's not hard. If you don't want to, I can do it." I started tearing up uncontrollably. The "it's not hard, I can do it" was meant kindly, but it stirred up a lot of feelings.

First, they didn't understand what needed to be asked when contacting a bakery for my allergy, so I'd have to instruct them on exactly what to say. Second, I usually prefer to email beforehand because I've found that establishments take more care in accuracy in their written responses. When I've called places, I've had instances where they reassured me over the phone, only for me to discover in person that they had overlooked something with my allergen. I find that over the phone people are often put on the spot and can forget critical details in their rush to give an answer.

Plus, I'd already reviewed the bakery's menu before our trip, which boasted new seasonal flavors weekly, so I wasn't hopeful that they could safely accommodate my needs. Of course, this was too much to put into words concisely, so I came off outwardly flustered. This story illustrates how one small comment can unearth a whirlwind of emotions, thoughts, and concerns for someone managing food allergies—issues that may not be immediately understood or visible to those without firsthand experience. I'm sure I could've taken deep breaths and acted more polite, but I wanted to share the real experience I had in a moment of distress and frustration.

Coping With a Lack of Labeling Law Protections

The lack of required, accurate, clear, and consistent food labeling laws in the US turns a grocery trip or online food order into a mental exercise in focus. Each label demands my full attention, as even the smallest detail can make a world of difference, and one wrong choice could lead to serious consequences. I've found that this scrutiny makes it difficult to focus on broader dietary goals as well.

So instead of noticing all the other nutritional details like exorbitant levels of saturated fat or sugar, my focus narrows to one key question: "Is it peanut-free or not?" Ensuring safety from a potentially life-or-death situation takes precedence over all else, highlighting the mental health impacts of our current US labeling, and emphasizing the anxiety and uncertainty it can cause. It's endless, as daily items like makeup, cleaning products, and even medications often contain hidden allergens. Without transparent labeling, it's difficult to determine what is safe.

The mental health impact of the combination of contamination risks and a lack of accommodations in public spaces cannot be overstated; it's a tough landscape to navigate. When food products are not labeled clearly, it can turn the most mundane meal into a guessing game. Additionally, public spaces like restaurants and schools frequently fall short of providing proper allergy accommodations.

If you didn't know it before reading this book, I hope you now see that having a food allergy is not just about avoiding the obvious allergens on an ingredient label or reading a restaurant menu. It's like weaving through a maze of uncertainties to uncover basic information while performing mental somersaults to live each day as safely as possible, all while managing the reality that much of the control we desire is beyond our reach.

I find myself endlessly analyzing each of the front-of-package marketing claims and sorting through misleading statements near the ingredients list, basically any time I grocery shop, and then again when re-checking the same items at home before eating them. Dining out can be equally tricky—reading and re-reading the description of dishes on the menu only to remember that details like the type of oils used and hidden proprietary seasonings aren't mentioned.

Seemingly safe foods can turn out to be dangerous in unexpected ways. With limited safe options, if I don't actively seek variety; my food choices can feel repetitive and plain. On the flip side, it means the world when a restaurant or brand is dedicated to being allergen-free or goes above and beyond to ensure their customers feel protected, comfortable, and able to eat safely.

Consider something as simple as a single French fry. For me, it quickly transforms into a puzzle. I find myself questioning the ingredients in the fryer oil, pondering what else has been cooked in that fryer, and whether my allergens might have been present during the cutting of the potato. I also wonder if the potato was grown in soil shared with peanuts, as the two are often cultivated together as companion plants. I'll question whether the person preparing my food had clean hands, and my inquiries quite literally can go on and on.

When I think about ordering a burger, the complexity only multiplies based on the plentiful opportunities for cross-contact. I do my best to find out about the source of the bun, asking whether allergens were processed in the same facility as it. Then there's the burger itself: *What's in it? What seasoning was used? Was it cooked in a contaminated pan?*

If it's a veggie burger made in-house of marinated carrots, sautéed beets, and black beans, my mind races to consider if the marinade is made in-house, and wondering about the sauteed vegetable oil. Even if the preparation was allergen-free, I think about the plate it's served on. If that plate came from a dishwasher that also cleaned peanut butter items, cross-contact could easily occur.

And I can't overlook the cheese and condiments. Which to me, are often most likely to come from facilities with my allergens. I often question whether the facility that sliced the cheese processes my allergens on shared equipment—most likely, I've learned from inquiring, they do. The same scrutiny applies to condiments, sauces, sides, and additional toppings. Every detail becomes a potential point of concern examined for cross-contact. Realistically, we all have to draw the line somewhere and learn to trust, and in my case, I take some comfort in knowing that I have epinephrine on hand if I need it.

The fact of the matter is that I usually can't know all the details. I may get some answers by asking the chef and kitchen staff questions, but there are limits to what restaurants can know and provide, especially regarding pre-packaged ingredients. They might have the product bottle on hand, but likely won't know the ins and outs of the allergens present in the bottling facility. They, too, are in the dark and lack the same knowledge of its sourcing and processing as the rest of consumers. I will place my order by factoring in all this to the best of my abilities, making them aware of my restrictions and needs.

These examples only scratch the surface of the daily mental load associated with managing food allergies while trying to stay safe in a world rife with contamination. It reminds me of a picture I shared on my social media platform and blog years ago—a grinder of sea salt with an ingredients label stating, "may contain soy." This highlights the uncertainty surrounding what's truly in our food. Most people remain unaware of these risks because allergens often aren't tracked or scrutinized to the extent necessary to avoid reactions.

Through the struggle to find safe food options, I've become more adept at finding workarounds. I've built a collection of favorite recipes, discovered places to eat that I trust asking about allergens, and continuously search for new products that suit my dietary needs. My partner, in-laws, and friends contribute by sharing recipes and safe food brands they find. It feels amazing to know others are thinking of me in this way, and I love finding new peanut-free products. To be honest, my options seem to be exponentially expanding compared to how things felt just a decade ago.

It's disheartening when a trusted product or brand becomes unsafe. In those moments, I often find myself grieving the realities of having a food allergy. It's particularly confusing when I experience a mild reaction—not requiring epinephrine but still needing antihistamines—to a brand that "should" be safe. If it's a one-off product that isn't a staple, I might let it go and not seek a replacement, and of course, if I reacted, I typically won't buy it again even if I've reached out to learn more.

However, if the product is a kitchen staple, I may enlist the help of someone I trust to find a suitable replacement or even create a safe version, which helps soften the blow of the change if I'm feeling particularly overwhelmed and can't do the research on my own. It's an emotional balancing act: I'm grateful for the expanding options and increasing food allergy awareness, yet I still feel the weight of each product that alters its practices.

If a product is no longer something I can eat due to ingredients, I make it a point to contact the company, expressing my sadness about the change and letting them know I won't be able to purchase their product(s) any longer. I let them know that I hope they track that feedback and understand the impact their decisions have on consumers like me.

Navigating Mental Health in Food Allergy Exposure Therapies

For individuals with food allergies, oral immunotherapy (OIT), tolerance induction programs (TIP), and similar exposure-based treatments are innovative but emotionally complex approaches. These therapies aim to increase a person's tolerance to allergens, yet they can be especially challenging for those with pre-existing behavioral health concerns. It's crucial to understand and address mental health as part of the preparation and process.

From my understanding, TIP is a more individualized approach compared with the standardized, templated OIT approach. It typically begins by introducing proteins that are similar to your allergens before gradually incorporating the allergen(s) themselves. This tailored method teaches the body to tolerate allergens and helps patients learn how to respond safely if a trigger occurs.

While TIP is not a cure, it can sometimes lead to a state of remission, where the immune system tolerates the allergens and reactions are minimized or eliminated. By the time you reach your specific allergens, you already have a base of tolerance from the earlier introduction of common proteins, making the process safer and more effective for managing multiple allergies.

For TIP specifically, there are currently no treatment options for patients over the age of 26. Those interested can register online to receive notifications if or when opportunities for older patients become available. Still, cost and location may make these therapies out of reach for many. Other options—such as EPIT (epicutaneous immunotherapy, typically delivered through a skin patch) and SLIT (sublingual immunotherapy, taken as drops or tablets under the tongue)—exist, but I hadn't even heard of them until I started attending food allergy conferences. That alone speaks volumes about the state of food allergy care in the US. Much of what I've learned has come from being part of the online allergy community and engaging with advocacy organizations—spaces that most people navigating a new diagnosis may not even know exist. We're simply not at the point yet where this kind of information is widely accessible to the general public, which is a reflection of how young and rapidly evolving the field still is.

Many individuals share their experiences online, and I highly recommend checking out allergy accounts to see firsthand what these therapies are like. From conversations I've had, some people with only one allergen often stick with avoidance, but those managing multiple allergens may seek TIP to gain additional tolerance. Otherwise, avoidance remains the primary "treatment option."

Balancing Readiness and Mental Health Needs

Therapies like OIT and TIP often require not only physical but also psychological readiness. For individuals with food allergies, therapy may be a necessary step before beginning treatment to build resilience and reduce anxiety. Collaborating with a psychologist skilled in food allergy-related trauma can help individuals and families navigate the stress of OIT. This is particularly important for children who may feel apprehensive or opposed to participating in food challenges, especially when parents prioritize the therapy.

Addressing Needle Phobia and Epinephrine Hesitancy

Needle phobia is a common barrier in food allergy treatment, especially when it involves the use of epinephrine injections. Exposure therapies can integrate gradual desensitization techniques to reduce the fear of needles, helping build confidence in using life-saving medication. This empowerment not only addresses phobias, but also enhances self-efficacy in managing allergic reactions. I am someone who does find needles intimidating, so I understand the hesitancy to use it immediately. The thought of injecting myself does give me pause, as I reach deep within myself to muster up the courage.

Assessing Risks and Limits Through Office-Based Exposure

Exposure therapy and cognitive-behavioral therapy (CBT) can be tailored to food allergy patients to assess and better understand their individual "thresholds" for airborne allergens or cross-contact risks. These sessions, conducted in controlled environments with a board-certified allergist, allow patients to explore their limits and risks safely. This personalized approach helps individuals and families make informed decisions about lifestyle adaptations and safety measures.

By combining exposure-based treatments with mental health strategies, patients can navigate these therapies with greater confidence, reducing the emotional toll of managing fatal allergies.

Navigating Safe Food Choices and Inflammation

Focusing on anti-inflammatory eating has become a key priority as I manage my autoimmune condition alongside my food allergy. I've set a goal to eat 30 different fruits and vegetables each week, which I recognize is a privilege to be able to do. The diversity in my diet not only helps my gut microbiome, but also encourages me to cut back on processed foods. To my surprise, it hasn't been as difficult as I expected, mostly because I've made a conscious effort to cram in as many varied ingredients wherever I can. Whether I'm tossing extra veggies into a salad, loading up different fruits into a smoothie, or preparing my overnight oats, I'm not being strict about it—it's just a goal I aim for. Over time, it has become more of a habit. It's less about perfection and more about intention.

If working with a dietitian or nutritionist is within reach, their guidance can be invaluable. However, it does require a certain level of education on labeling laws and my food allergy experience, since it isn't common knowledge. Even so, I've benefited immensely from their expertise, gaining confidence in my food choices and learning how to make beneficial eating habits stick. They've also helped save time finding alternatives to substitutes in recipes, which is valuable when you're already spending hours researching safe food and non-food items on a regular basis. But if working with someone is an option, there are so many free, fantastic resources out there. I've had great success discovering nutritious and tasty recipes on my own through trial and error, looking online, and even gaining inspiration from books at my public library.

While there can be an overwhelming amount of information when it comes to free recipes online, I find it helpful to focus on recipes with lots of positive reviews and high ratings of 4-5 stars. Between these resources and a bit of experimentation, I've gained more confidence in crafting meals that are safe, anti-inflammatory, and enjoyable. That said, sourcing safe food items can still be tricky. Due to that, I tend to stick with familiar raw, single-ingredient products and make many meals from scratch. While it can be limiting, it also provides a sense of control in a world where my food safety is never guaranteed.

In case you're looking to focus on anti-inflammatory eating, my biggest takeaway is this: prioritize whole, unprocessed foods when possible. Coincidentally, this is the same approach I take when I'm frustrated by the lack of safe, peanut-free products. In those moments, I shift my focus to simple, whole-ingredient meals from the produce section—it's a way to regain control and simplify the process. Meals like roasted vegetables paired with a fresh salad drizzled with my homemade dressing, and for snacks, I may opt for thoroughly washed chopped veggies or fruit. It's also worth looking up foods that are naturally anti-inflammatory and working those in if you can.

This relentless cycle of searching, planning, and ultimately feeling limited can take a toll on my mental well-being, especially when other life stressors are in play. This type of stress can quickly cause a ripple effect, creating an even heavier burden. I hope this serves as a reminder of the continual vigilance required to navigate a world where food safety is often uncertain.

On my website I explore the nuanced ways I cope with and navigate hyper-specific situations, such as staying in hotels, attending weddings, or going to the gym—a place filled with protein snacks and meals containing my allergens. With this foundation laid, let's dive into the coping strategies I regularly use. Keep in mind that these approaches work for me; I'm sharing them not as strict advice, but in the hopes that they may provide support or inspire ideas for you, too.

Living Mindfully

I've likened living with food allergies to an emotional rollercoaster, with high highs and low lows. Incorporating mindfulness and stress management techniques that resonate with you into your daily or weekly routine can be incredibly beneficial for navigating these fluctuating emotions we must manage. While committing to a daily practice is a challenge for me, I strive to make it a goal, aiming to engage in mindfulness exercises a few times a week. Though, on particularly stressful days, I may turn to these practices multiple times.

The term mindfulness involves staying present and fully engaging with the current moment. This practice can allow you to observe your thoughts and feelings without judgment, helping you cultivate a sense of calm in your mind and body. One simple way to practice mindfulness is through breathing exercises. I often will simply take a few breaths, making sure my exhales are longer than my inhales. It doesn't have to be anything formal, but taking a few moments each day to focus on your breath can be enough to ground you.

I often catch myself mid-workday, realizing that my breathing has become tight and shallow. In those moments, I take a few moments for a quick breathing exercise and can literally feel the shift in my heartbeat, stepping out of that fight-or-flight mode. I don't even need to get up from my desk; I practice this while working, shopping, or sitting in my car. I truly believe that everyone can benefit from conscious breathing. If you want to give it a try, inhale for a count of four, hold for four, and exhale for eight. This rhythmic breathing can help center your thoughts, especially when you're feeling overwhelmed.

Not only does practicing meditation loosen up the tension I tend to hold in my body, but it also helps take my anxiety and racing mind down multiple notches to a more manageable place. If you haven't tried them yet, guided meditations focused on anxiety reduction or visualizations that promote a sense of safety and control can be incredibly helpful. Apps like Headspace or Calm offer a variety of options tailored to different needs and levels of experience, but I've also listened to some free ones on YouTube.

I've also come across a lot of research about the benefits of forest bathing and spending time in nature for both mental well-being and physical health, like lowering blood pressure and reducing the risk of cardiovascular disease and diabetes. Forest bathing, known as "Shinrin-yoku" in Japanese, has been extensively studied in Japan, with findings showing that even a walk in a busy city will provide more mental and physical benefits compared to staying indoors—where we spend about 90% of our lives according to the US Environmental Protection Agency's *A Guide to Indoor Air Quality*.

This finding is reassuring to me, especially knowing that just walking through my city neighborhood, which has some greenery but also plenty of concrete and noise, still helps calm my nervous system. I've always felt better after spending time outdoors, so I make it a point to expose myself to the elements year-round, no matter the season.

While I try to go hiking whenever I can, I've discovered that sitting outside with a book, lying back and watching the clouds drift by, or taking a gentle walk while being mindful of my surroundings are more easily attainable options. As a result, I'm able to incorporate those activities into my routine more often than a full hike. A recent Kaiser article on forest bathing found that spending just 10 to 20 minutes a day outdoors can lead to increased happiness and decreased stress, which gives me hope since it's not a significant outdoor investment.

And while speaking of mindfulness, I can't discuss it without mentioning yoga. There are many styles of yoga, all of which combine physical movements—easily adapted for anyone—and breath awareness. Yoga not only promotes physical health and flexibility but also alleviates stress and anxiety through breathwork and mental focus. Simple poses, like child's pose, butterfly pose, legs-up-the-wall pose, or downward dog (along with their modifications), can encourage relaxation. I find that attending classes keeps me motivated and engaged throughout the session, while at home, my mind tends to wander more, and I may rush through the routine and end up doing my own shortened version. Regardless, some yoga and stretching are surely better than none!

A Harvard health study on yoga's mental health benefits highlights that yoga goes beyond physical exercise, offering significant mental health advantages:

- Yoga strengthens brain connections and improves cognitive skills like learning and memory, regular practice can lead to a thicker cerebral cortex and hippocampus.
- Elevates gamma-aminobutyric acid (GABA), a brain chemical associated with improved mood and reduced anxiety.
- Reduces emotional reactivity by decreasing activity in the limbic system.

  WebMD reports that yoga can release mood-boosting brain

chemicals like dopamine, serotonin, and norepinephrine. Simply put, incorporating any of the mindfulness practices I've mentioned here can help empower you to manage the physical and emotional toll of living with or managing food allergies. These research-backed strategies are designed to help you face daily challenges with greater ease and confidence.

Workplace Accommodations

Now, let's switch gears and talk about managing food allergies in the workplace, an environment where accommodations can significantly shape not only your day-to-day experience, but also the trajectory of your career. Even though it was over a decade ago, I can still vividly remember passing by my previous employer's large glass wall looking into the breakroom, and seeing most of my department gathered for lunch, joyfully chatting and bonding. Meanwhile, I was on the other side of the glass, in the hallway, wishing I could join in. I couldn't because of my peanut allergy and a lack of accommodations at my workplace. This particular employer had prohibited peanut ingredients in my specific wing of the building, but this didn't extend to the breakroom. Plus, I was responsible for letting my "wing" know and enforcing it.

As a result, I frequently missed out on opportunities to connect with colleagues, build friendships, and foster important networking relationships—all of which play a huge role in professional development. I hated that I had to avoid the social camaraderie that comes with communal meals. I'd try eating outside on our shared patio off the kitchen sometimes with others when it was nice weather, only to catch a whiff of peanuts and have to scurry away mid-conversation in fear.

The reality was, most days I found myself eating at my desk, occasionally switching it up to sit in my car, even on extreme weather days when it was sweltering hot or freezing cold. I felt stuck, glued to the building, and sometimes just needed to get out.

I could only bring room-temperature foods to work since I had no access to a fridge or microwave without risking exposure to peanuts in the break room. I craved the warmth of hot meals, or better yet, the opportunity to partake in the free unsafe meals often provided by my employer.

Reflecting on my time there from 2008 to 2013, I realize how much I missed out on both in building relationships and larger workplace opportunities. These missed connections highlight how powerful all accommodations are for inclusion, not just for safety but also for fostering meaningful professional relationships, career opportunities, and more.

This sense of isolation is amplified by broader societal misunderstandings about food allergies, too. As I touched on in the previous chapter, the 2024 Super Bowl commercial making light of anaphylaxis highlights not only the broader societal misunderstandings about food allergies, but also how far we still have to go in terms of awareness—whether in the workplace or elsewhere.

These inaccurate attempts at comedic food allergy portrayals reinforce the lack of empathy and awareness we often face in professional environments. They mirror the challenges experienced in many workplaces, where food allergies can be trivialized or misunderstood, leading to inadequate accommodations and an environment where those with allergies feel marginalized and excluded. Witnessing such insensitivity—whether directly, through media, or second hand—intensifies the emotional strain we endure. And this doesn't even address the physical toll of allergic reactions and the lingering effects that can persist for days, weeks, or even for life.

Take the case of Amy May Shead, a thriving 26-year-old UK resident whose life was forever altered in 2014 after suffering a catastrophic allergic reaction while dining out in Budapest. Despite providing her allergy information card, printed in the local language, to inform the restaurant of her nut allergy, she experienced anaphylaxis followed by cardiac arrest.

As a result, Amy now lives with a neuro-disability and can't live independently. Her story is a heartbreaking reminder of how serious food allergies are. You can learn more about her journey and the incredible advocacy work of her loved ones through the Amy May Trust, which continues to raise awareness about the severity of food allergies and their life-altering impacts.

The traumatisms we face in the food allergy space can often be categorized as both "big T" trauma, like life-threatening allergic reactions, and "little t" trauma, such as the daily stress of navigating a world that frequently dismisses our experiences. After facing these hurdles myself, I sought solace in exploring the intersection of food allergies and mental health, normalizing experiences that, until recently, I rarely saw discussed.

Self-Compassion and Acceptance

Living with food allergies comes with many unique challenges, so being kind to yourself and acknowledging that it's okay to feel frustrated, sad, jealous, resentful, guilty, and any other emotions that may come up for you. It is, I've found, a normal part of food allergy life. Accepting the realities of your situation doesn't mean that you're giving in to fear or that you're weak; instead, it means healthily recognizing your feelings and allowing yourself to process them.

Celebrate your strengths and achievements, no matter how small they may seem, and emphasize self-compassion when needed. I truly believe that self-acceptance and self-love can empower you to navigate your food allergy journey with greater adaptability and resilience, whether you are a food allergy parent, an individual with food allergies, or someone impacted in another way.

One funny encounter I had at a Courage at Congress event hosted by FARE a few years ago has stuck with me, bringing a smile to my face whenever I think of it. I struck up a conversation with a food allergy mom while we were practicing getting ready to talk to our state representatives. Her daughter, who was about eight years old, had been born with allergies. Before this experience, the mom had little awareness of food allergies, but after eight years of practice, she had become an avid food allergy expert in ways she never imagined she would be.

As she shared a story about the guilt she sometimes felt regarding her daughter's allergies, she mentioned, "I'm a worrier." I misheard her and exclaimed back enthusiastically, "You *ARE* a warrior!" while placing my hand on her shoulder and smiling proudly. She laughed and clarified her comment. We both agreed that she was indeed both—a worrier and a food allergy warrior. And that I am, too.

Fostering and maintaining a positive outlook despite the challenges of living with food allergies is a constant practice, but it's one I'm committed to because I know it's worth it. I enjoy engaging in activities that uplift my spirits, and I encourage you to do the same. Surround yourself with compassionate people, pursue hobbies you love, and practice experiencing joy.

Focusing on what you can control and celebrating small victories along the way has significantly impacted my mental wellness. By adopting a positive and creative mindset that's tailored to you, you can empower yourself to face challenges with optimism and ingenuity, allowing you to lead a fulfilling life even in the face of dietary restrictions.

According to a study by Teresa Amabile from Harvard Business School, people who tracked their small achievements every day enhanced their motivation. This simple practice of recording progress helps boost confidence and releases dopamine, which improves mood, motivation, and attention. Additional research shows that experiencing positive emotions not only increases momentary happiness but also helps develop qualities like optimism and resilience, which can protect against distress and poor mental health in the future. Engaging in small "micro-joys" daily has the potential to elevate both short- and long-term mental health.

For those living with chronic conditions, appreciating simple pleasures can be particularly impactful. Small joys can enhance daily life and general well-being, helping to maintain a positive outlook, despite ongoing challenges.

By focusing on what you can control and regularly celebrating small wins, you're employing evidence-based strategies that can significantly impact mental wellness. Letting each win matter is especially important when managing the complexities of food allergies.

As we transition into the next section, we'll further explore the importance of having social support systems to enhance your well-being and provide a meaningful sense of community. I saw a quote recently shared around the food allergy community that resonated; it went something like, "Your circle should want you to win, and your circle should clap the loudest when you have good news. If they don't, find a new circle." In the spirit of following that advice, let's talk about support networks.

Strength in Support

Living with a food allergy presents unique challenges, but having a strong community to fall back on can transform the experience into something exponentially more manageable.

Support goes beyond practical assistance; it includes emotional understanding, empathy, and the freedom to be your authentic self without fear of judgment. Having access to this provides an invisible sense of security, helping you navigate the complexities of daily life with food allergies and beyond.

In this section, we'll delve into the profound impact of therapy, which can provide essential emotional relief and the importance of connecting with others both online and offline.

We'll also discuss the value of cultivating a close-knit network of people who genuinely care about your wellbeing on your journey—and whom you can lift up in return. Whether through professional guidance, understanding colleagues, or meaningful friendships, these connections can be life-changing and transformative, allowing them to be their authentic selves. Fostering these close-knit relationships, whether virtual or in-person, can make navigating life with food allergies—or any challenge—a little easier.

A study published in the 2024 journal *Frontiers in Psychology* provides evidence for the mental health benefits of social support. The research found:

- Higher levels of social support are associated with lower rates of depression, anxiety, and stress.

- Social support significantly shapes how individuals perceive and handle stress, acting as a crucial resource when facing challenges.

- A robust support system can alleviate the overwhelming nature of specific events, contributing to better mental health outcomes.

The study, anchored in Lazarus and Folkman's stress and coping theory, highlights that social support is a pivotal factor influencing how individuals perceive and manage stress, consequently impacting mental health.

I recall a quote from bell hooks' book, *All About Love*, that a best friend shared with me in conversation years ago that emphasizes that friendship can be as transformative and impactful as romantic relationships, or even more so. Much of bell hooks's writing suggests that a meaningful friendship is one of the most radical connections a person can have, characterized by openness, vulnerability, and mutual growth. Since meaningful friendships involve intimacy, trust, and understanding, they challenge societal norms and foster personal development in ways similar to romantic love. By being open with a friend, individuals can gain valuable insights and work toward personal growth in ways we may not glean from a romantic partner.

It's clear that living with food allergies goes beyond the physical challenges linked to the body's immune response; it significantly affects mental well-being and daily life. One of the emotional burdens I face the most is the sense of restriction. I frequently find myself wishing I could eat as freely as others do—choosing foods based solely on convenience, taste, and preferences. Instead, my choices are largely determined by what is least likely to trigger an allergic response, pushing taste and convenience to the backseat.

While formal therapy with a licensed provider offers a safe space to explore and manage the trauma, stress, anxiety, and frustration that often accompany chronic conditions, support groups can also fulfill a unique role. They allow individuals to share personal experiences with others who truly "get it," providing a sense of validation and understanding. This communal sharing not only fosters emotional strength but also encourages practical coping strategies as members gain insights from others facing similar challenges in ways a trained therapist may not be able to provide without first-hand experience.

Community Connections

The importance of community for individuals with chronic conditions is well-documented in research. The same *Frontiers in Psychology* journal highlights several key benefits of support groups for those managing chronic illnesses such as improved disease management, emotional validation, enhanced access to resources, cost-effectiveness, and practical coping strategies.

For the past couple years I've been organizing a free, inclusive meetup called the Inclusive Allergy and Autoimmune Meetup (IAAM) in Louisville, where individuals with allergies or autoimmune issues can come together to chat and share experiences. I co-lead this initiative with another member of the food allergy and autoimmune community, a specialty diet and allergy chef, which helps alleviate the pressure on both of us in case one of us gets sick or has a flare-up. Knock on wood, we haven't had to cancel any meetings yet, and we both attended each session for over the first year, providing a compassionate connection to everyone who can join us in person.

One of our regular attendees said our meetups feel akin to an Alcoholics Anonymous (AA) meeting and even suggested that we hold them twice a month instead of our current monthly schedule. He shared that attending these meetups helps him feel less isolated and alone, and he leaves feeling mentally uplifted. I can relate to this sentiment; I've always felt better after our meetups, too. There's something incredibly refreshing about being in a room full of people who understand your experiences without the need for extensive explanations about your symptoms. It creates a collective bond that is nearly impossible to find elsewhere, transcending age, gender, and other typical physical differences.

Due to our time limits, we haven't been offering online versions of our meetups because similar groups already exist across the US and globally. Our focus has been on finding mutual connections in our local region. If you're looking to join a group, I encourage you to explore the online options available. Additionally, if you're inspired to create your free meetup, I've shared resources on my website and social media about how we run ours. It's held in a public space that costs us nothing except for the time we dedicate to it. My resources are freely available for anyone to use to establish an allergy and autoimmune group or any kind of community they wish to create.

Building a supportive network is helpful for finding that needed sense of belonging, shared experiences, and security for any type of difficulty in life, food allergies, or other. Both online and offline communities can play a role in this, as online meetups offer accessibility to resources and friends from around the globe, while local in-person interactions can provide more tangible location-specific assistance.

Finding Your People

Surrounding yourself with people who genuinely care, listen, and encourage you is indispensable. True friends will respect your dietary needs, help you navigate social situations, and provide empathy during both the ups and downs. It's equally important to establish healthy boundaries with those who dismiss or trivialize your food allergy concerns.

If you already have a circle of friends like this, that's amazing! However, as time goes on, friendships can shift, and distances can grow, making it essential to know how to build a genuine community anew. Cultivating relationships that uplift and empower you can take time and may evolve, but doing so significantly alleviates the daily challenges of managing food allergies, ultimately creating a safer and more enjoyable life.

Finding your best friend group often starts with identifying those who genuinely care about you. I focus on surrounding myself with people I can truly be myself around, and I consciously invest my energy in nurturing those relationships. It's about creating a circle that fosters mutual understanding and shared experiences. It doesn't matter how I meet them; it could be at a local event, through a mutual friend, from a colleague, or even by complimenting someone in passing and striking up a conversation. Each interaction has the potential to lead to meaningful connections that enrich our lives.

By focusing on nurturing connections that offer mutual love and care, I can create an environment where I feel valued and safe, allowing me to navigate life with food allergies more confidently. It's about surrounding yourself with friends who not only accept your dietary boundaries but also celebrate your uniqueness and want to be in your corner cheering you on, making the journey of managing food allergies a shared experience rather than a solitary one.

Eating out at a restaurant with a large group of others with food allergies is something I've only experienced recently, in my mid-thirties. When the stars aligned and I finally got together in person with some people I'd met virtually, it was incredibly fun and healing. Affirming, normalized, refreshing—*all* the things. Everyone knew how to use an epi, understood the experience and the fears, and without even needing to say it, offered genuine support. I highly recommend meeting your food allergy friends in real life if that's something you think you might enjoy. It's a special kind of community that helps lessen the isolation many of us feel.

Since anyone can develop an allergy, or disability, or go through significant life transitions at any time, it's all about finding others who understand and genuinely want to accommodate and be there for their friends and family. Connection is one of my core values and so I deeply appreciate genuineness and emotional vulnerability in my relationships. When I share my experiences with those who truly listen and see me, and vice versa, it facilitates a sense of community that helps alleviate the weight of whatever it is I'm going through. It's comforting to know I'm not alone in navigating these challenges, and it reinforces the idea that we can show up for each other through our individual journeys even if we aren't experiencing the exact same thing.

While engaging with a community about allergies offers numerous benefits—like raising awareness and building connections—being a blogger and active on social media can sometimes be draining and discouraging. The constant pressure to create content, keep up with trends, and interact with followers can take a toll on mental well-being. Balancing the desire to share valuable information with the need for self-care is essential. Unfortunately, advocating online can lead to rude comments, demands from the same community you're trying to help, and a significant amount of unwanted negativity.

The 2024 *Frontiers in Psychology* journal also investigated the impact of popularity on the mental health of social media influencers. The study revealed that an increase in the number of followers was associated with increased negative emotions.

This suggests that as an influencer's audience grows, so does the potential for mental health challenges, possibly due to increased pressure and exposure to negative feedback.

Interestingly, the research found that influencers earning less than $10,000 from social media reported the lowest negative feeling scores. This could indicate that those who are less financially dependent on their social media presence may experience less pressure and stress. A study published in the American Marketing Association's 2024 *Journal of Marketing* found that influencers who disable social media comments are perceived as less sincere and ultimately incur both interpersonal and professional consequences. This puts influencers in a difficult position, as leaving comments open can expose them to negativity, but disabling them can harm their perceived authenticity and connection with followers. This research supports the importance of prioritizing self-care and mental well-being while navigating the demands of online advocacy and engagement.

There are moments when I need to step back and take a breather from my advocate role—not just online, but also in real life. Navigating food allergy accommodations and conversations face-to-face can feel much more personal and mentally exhausting, making it important that I prioritize my own well-being first.

For instance, I might choose to leave a local venue that isn't accommodating rather than try to convince them to make adjustments if I'm feeling low on energy. Recently, I attended a concert with a friend and saw people walking toward us carrying king-sized boxes of peanut M&Ms.

My friend noticed my distress and quickly offered to speak to them, since we knew they were about to sit in the two open seats next to us, and asked if they would mind moving elsewhere to eat due to my airborne allergy. I felt an immense sense of relief wash over me as I exclaimed, "YES, PLEASE! THANK YOU!!" It felt like a huge weight had been lifted off my shoulders, allowing me to enjoy the moment without the mental strain of initiating that conversation and worrying about how the two women might respond. At that moment, I didn't feel weak or ashamed—I just felt grateful for my friend.

I know I've done the same for friends who have been too anxious to ask for something; I may step up and ask on their behalf. It goes both ways. It's a beautiful reminder of how mutual support strengthens our friendships and benefits our lives in ways beyond what we may even immediately recognize.

While many public interactions I've had have been positive, the unpredictability of how conversations might unfold—especially with the potential for confusion, being disregarded, or rudeness—can be daunting. Having others advocate for me in certain environments, help me find a safe product when I feel overwhelmed, is deeply appreciated. I can do life completely independently, but it's nice having others I trust who want to care for me in this way.

For instance, at family events on my husband's side, I often rely on him to handle discussions about my food allergy. This allows me to navigate these situations with less anxiety. Given that I routinely manage conversations with restaurants, brands, friends, family, and workplaces about my allergies, asking for his assistance in these instances feels like a well-deserved break. It often feels more appropriate coming from him, and I genuinely appreciate his help. He's happy to step in, which makes navigating these situations much easier for me.

Divvying up the work, whenever possible, and finding opportunities to pause in advocating for your needs is something I highly recommend. Consider how you can incorporate these pockets of rest into your life, even if it's only a few times a year, to give yourself the much-deserved break where you don't have to *do* and can just *be*. These pauses remind us that we're human beings, not only defined by constant doing.

Building a Network for Emergencies

Preparing for potential allergic reactions is a major part of living with food allergies, but it doesn't have to be a solo effort. While it's essential to always carry your epinephrine and other prescribed emergency medications, it's equally important to ensure they are easily accessible and that those around you know where they're located. Creating a clear allergy action plan can take many forms. For example, you might provide a verbal reminder at the start of an event to a select few you trust or create a written outline detailing the steps to take during a reaction, displayed in a public space or passed out on paper for others to keep on hand. Sharing your emergency plan with friends, family, teachers, employers, and colleagues helps build a reliable network, ensuring they feel confident assisting you.

Educating the people in your life about your specific allergens and how to respond in the event of anaphylaxis or a milder allergic reaction not only safeguards your well-being but also creates trust. This proactive approach can alleviate anxiety and worry for all involved.

Empowering others to participate in your preparedness creates a safety net that can significantly reduce stress during an emergency, ensuring you receive the right care as quickly as possible. Additionally, it prepares those around you to act confidently in case they witness someone else experiencing anaphylaxis, or even face a reaction themselves, equipping them with the basics of what to do.

Something I need to do more often, is show friends, family, colleagues, and anyone I'm with regularly how to administer my medications. Some medications even come with a "trainer," which is great for getting a hands-on feel for what to do in real-life situations. The truth is, the more we get comfortable taking up a little time and educating our circles, the better we all are for it.

It's not selfish to train others on how to use your medications, this knowledge comes in handy for so many situations and could benefit many others in times of need.

Advocating For Your Needs in the Real World

Advocating for yourself—or having someone advocate for you—can be very helpful when managing food allergies or conditions like celiac disease or eosinophilic esophagitis (EoE). If you don't know how, start by clearly communicating your needs and writing those out if you feel unsure how you want to phrase them. I've read line by line from my Notes app on my phone because I knew the moment I asked in person I'd feel nervous and potentially get my request jumbled up or I'd forget to ask something.

If it's at a restaurant, don't hesitate to ask specific questions about ingredients and preparation. For example, I always ask about peanut ingredients in dishes like mole sauce or chili, at the bar, in desserts, or on their kid's menu, because I know those are commonly overlooked spots to find peanuts, and it helps open the conversation into more of a discussion and exchange of information and understanding.

When in doubt, if you feel your needs are unresolved, it's always worth asking extra questions. If their answers still leave you without the clarity or understanding you hoped for, remember that you don't have to eat someplace if you're uncomfortable. When I find a place that's thorough and transparent in their replies and willing to go into detail, they become a place I tend to reach out to when we want to safely dine out. I never try to force a place into being that way—it must come naturally and with a desire for safety from their end.

When advocating for accommodations in school settings, providing teachers, professors, and other staff, such as counselors or HR, with an allergy action plan can help get your exact needs met. Even better, you can likely formulate the action plan with them, bouncing back and forth so the results have clear expectations.

Lastly, consider sharing articles or resources that resonate with your personal experiences regarding food allergies to help others better understand. If you find a particular book insightful—like, oh I don't know, this one perhaps (just saying!) you might suggest it by expressing, "I think you might enjoy this—it offers a deeper understanding of the food allergy experience." This approach allows you to provide an opportunity for learning without putting pressure on them and saves you from having to do all the explaining yourself. However, if they choose not to read it, I've found that can sometimes be disappointing. That said, nothing beats one-on-one conversations where you can use examples from your own life to convey the specific points you want others to grasp about your experience on the allergy reactivity spectrum.

Media's Influence on Mental Health

The way the media portrays food allergies, disabilities, and any marginalized population exceedingly influences public perception, individual mental health, and public bias. Understandably, negative media representations of food allergies can exacerbate the existing mental health issues of those experiencing or managing them. A content analysis published in the PubMed journal *Health Communication* found that food allergies in entertainment media were most frequently portrayed in a humorous context and often contained inaccurate information. A follow-up experiment in the same study showed that viewing humorous portrayals of food allergies had an indirect negative effect on health policy support by decreasing the perceived seriousness of food allergies.

When serious conditions are inaccurately portrayed or stigmatized, they further alienate affected communities, making it more difficult for those outside their experiences to develop empathy and understanding. This dual nature of media influence underscores the importance of accurate and positive representation.

As a result, I advocate for directly consulting the communities being depicted to ensure their voices and perspectives are respected and portrayed authentically.

Negative portrayals of food allergies in media can perpetuate harmful stereotypes and significantly increase the emotional burden for those affected. Misrepresentation can lead to heightened anxiety and feelings of isolation among individuals managing food allergies. Conversely, positive and accurate representations play a crucial role in alleviating stigma and fostering empathy. A study by FARE concluded that participants exposed to humorous portrayals of food allergies were more likely to have negative attitudes toward those with food allergies, perceive food allergies as less serious, and be less likely to take life-saving measures in an emergency.

When food allergies and disabilities are displayed with sensitivity, it not only educates the public but also promotes compassion, creating a more inclusive society where individuals feel seen and validated. Media can evoke a range of emotions—humor, joy, sorrow, or desire—while remaining respectful. Studies demonstrate that positive representation empowers those living with these conditions by correctly depicting their experiences and challenges, ultimately helping to build an empathetic environment for all. It's essential to understand how both the external world, like the media, and our internal experiences contribute to this complex reality.

Reducing The Stigma

I've come to understand the profound impact stigma has on our lives, especially when it comes to "invisible disabilities" like mental health conditions or food allergies. The stigma surrounding invisible disabilities, including mental health conditions and food allergies, is indeed prevalent and impactful as a recent 2023 ReThink survey revealed, three in five people (58%) living with a mental illness did not seek help due to concerns about how they would be perceived by others. An American Medical ID survey found that 96% of people with chronic health conditions have an invisible illness, which can lead to stigma and discrimination in various aspects of life, including relationships, education, healthcare, and employment.

These internal struggles often go unseen, leading to misunderstandings, disbelief, and judgment from others. When people can't visibly see a challenge, they're less likely to acknowledge its reality. That's why the name *Invisibly Allergic* came to be—to shed light on the hidden, often misunderstood realities of living with life-threatening food allergies. Considering mental health within the framework of disability rights is fundamental. Just as we advocate for physical accommodations and support, ensuring access to mental health care and accommodations is equally vital. Mental health issues are legitimate disabilities that deserve understanding, validation, and acting proactively—not discrimination.

The stigma surrounding mental health doesn't exist in isolation—it intersects with other forms of discrimination, such as race, gender, and socioeconomic status. These overlapping factors create differing challenges for individuals who face multiple forms of marginalization. Access to proper healthcare can vary dramatically depending on someone's background or financial situation, compounding the effects of both mental health stigma and food allergy management. Addressing stigma involves recognizing and dismantling these interconnected inequities, while encouraging a broad spectrum of inclusivity for everyone, regardless of their identity or circumstances.

So, what can we do? Advocacy and education are two of the most powerful tools we have to combat stigma. By advocating for mental health to be recognized as a legitimate part of the disability spectrum, we can foster greater acceptance within our communities. Education about mental health helps dismantle misconceptions and fears, making room for welcoming environments where individuals feel safe to seek help without judgment.

Many people still don't fully understand mental health conditions, often viewing them as signs of weakness or personal failings, rather than as genuine medical concerns that deserve attention and care. An NIMH article explains how in 2022, among the 59.3 million adults with Any Mental Illness (AMI) in the US, only 50.6% received mental health treatment in the past year.

Cultural beliefs can sometimes complicate the landscape of mental health stigma in diverse ways, too. In many regions, mental health struggles are still viewed as taboo and directly associated with shame. These norms can hinder individuals from seeking help or even discussing their experiences openly, leading to continued silence and isolation. Moreover, these societal attitudes often lead to self-stigma, where individuals internalize negative perceptions, feeling ashamed or guilty about their condition. This internal conflict can erode self-esteem and hinder access to healing. Bias and stigma surrounding mental health can vary widely across cultures and regions, underscoring the need for tailored advocacy and education.

By promoting a compassionate understanding of mental health as an essential aspect of human diversity and addressing the roots of stigma—be it historical, cultural, or media-driven—we can foster communities where everyone feels valued, regardless of their mental health or mental illness challenges.

Suicide Prevention

If you or someone you know is struggling with thoughts of suicide, please seek help immediately. As someone who has lost a dear friend far too young to suicide, this issue is deeply personal to me. You are not alone, and I promise help is within reach.

Reducing the stigma surrounding suicide is crucial for creating an environment where individuals feel safe to share their struggles without fear of judgment or burdening others. Open and honest conversations about mental health and suicide can provide much-needed support and foster understanding.

As someone who has personally experienced depression and suicidal thoughts, I want to share this to help normalize these conversations in the world we live in. Having these thoughts doesn't mean you have to give up or feel shame. There is hope, and reaching out for help is a powerful step. For reliable statistics on the crossover between mental health and food allergies, consider these reputable sources:

1. *American Academy of Allergy, Asthma & Immunology (AAAAI)*

AAAAI offers comprehensive information on food allergies, including prevalence, symptoms, and management, all backed by scientific research. They provide valuable resources for both patients and healthcare providers, ensuring that individuals have access to the latest information and treatment guidelines.

2. *Centers for Disease Control and Prevention (CDC)*

The CDC presents data on the prevalence of food allergies in the US, alongside related health issues and demographic statistics. Their resources aim to inform public health initiatives and promote awareness about food allergies, contributing to better understanding and management of these conditions.

3. *Food Allergy & Anaphylaxis Connection Team (FAACT)*

FAACT offers a wealth of free educational resources and advocacy support for individuals managing food allergies. Their comprehensive Behavioral Health Resource Center specifically addresses the mental health aspects related to food allergies, providing guidance on coping skills, resilience building, and managing anxiety and depression. Beyond behavioral health, FAACT's other resource centers—covering Education in Schools, Civil Rights Advocacy, and Inclusion Initiatives—offer additional tools and support that intersect with emotional well-being, helping individuals and families manage both the practical and psychological aspects of food allergies.

4. *Center for Food Allergy & Asthma Research (CFAAR)*

CFAAR is dedicated to conducting research on food allergies and asthma, delivering insights into their prevalence, causes, and treatment through scientific studies and public health initiatives. The center places a strong emphasis on mental health, focusing on the psychological impact of food allergies and providing guidance and resources for individuals coping with these challenges.

5. *PubMed (NIH)*

PubMed, maintained by the National Institutes of Health, serves as a crucial resource for accessing a vast database of scientific literature on all types of topics, including food allergies and mental health intersections. With some digging and searching, users can find valuable research on the mental health implications of living with food allergies, as well as insights into coping mechanisms and strategies.

Dealing with Food Allergy Bullies

When I think about food allergy bullying, my mind inevitably returns to that moment in high school with Alana—the friend who handed me her Reese's Puffs cereal to try, knowing full well it contained peanuts. That betrayal carved a permanent mark in my memory, not only because it put my life at risk, but because it left me questioning what I thought was a close friendship. Experiences like that remind me that food allergy bullying isn't abstract; it's real, it's personal, and its impact lasts long after the moment passes.

Dealing with food allergy bullying is challenging and

can be emotionally draining. It's not just hurtful comments; the consequences can be serious and even life-threatening, like anaphylaxis. The worry about being bullied while monitoring for a potential allergic reaction can leave people feeling isolated and anxious. The impact isn't just in the moment; it's the lasting uncertainty, the way it makes you question who you can trust. First and foremost, it's important to remember that you are not alone in facing this issue; finding solidarity in this can hopefully provide some sense of empowerment. When confronted with any type of bullying, I've learned that prioritizing the safety and well-being of the bullied individual should always be the top concern and first order of business.

Here are some practical tips and strategies I've gathered from my own experiences to help you handle and cope with these unfortunate encounters that might come up—hopefully not, but you never know. While these insights come from my journey, I'm not a mental health professional.

- Setting Boundaries and Prioritizing Safety: While assertive communication can be effective, it's okay to set clear boundaries if you're feeling emotional or prefer not to engage directly. This might involve removing yourself from the situation, seeking help from a teacher, colleague, friend, or supervisor, and avoiding interactions where your allergens aren't taken seriously. Your primary goal is to protect yourself, so prioritize your emotional well-being in however you respond.

- Seeking Assistance: Lean on trusted friends, family members, or community groups who understand your situation. These people can offer emotional validation and practical advice for managing challenging interactions that may fall under bullying.

- Education and Awareness: If the bullying feels more like ignorance than malice, and you're up for it, consider taking the opportunity to educate others about food allergies and the serious risks involved. Sometimes, bullying comes from misunderstanding rather than bad intentions. By sharing what you know, you can help build understanding among your peers and the community. I'm always amazed by friends who are great communicators—they often find common ground with others in ways I never thought possible.

- Document Incidents: Make sure to keep a written record of any bullying incidents, noting the dates, locations, and what happened. This documentation can be super helpful if you choose to report the bullying to someone in authority or need extra support later. I've learned from experience that if incidents happen months apart, it's easy to forget the details, which can mess up the timeline you want to present when seeking help.

- Professional Help: Think about reaching out to a mental health professional who understands the trauma or stress of living with chronic health issues. They can offer strategies to help you manage anxiety, build resilience, and handle unfortunate social situations. Remember, the bullying isn't your fault.

More Than Just Words

Food allergy bullying can be different from other types of bullying because it's about allergens and the real risk of physical harm. This kind of bullying can lead to medical emergencies and, sadly, even death. It's important for us as a society to understand the emotional impact that this kind of bullying can have.

Getting assistance from a therapist or doctor can be important if you're dealing with a bully, as mental health is just as important as physical health. Here are the key ways food allergy bullying stands out as a unique issue. I point this out because it may be overlooked and can require specific attention and handling:

- Uniqueness of Trigger: Food allergy bullying involves targeting someone based on their dietary restrictions or allergies. Unlike other forms of bullying that may focus on personal attributes or characteristics, food allergy bullying revolves around the specific allergens that can cause severe physical harm from allergic reactions. The same applies to other similar conditions, like celiac disease, EoE, FPIES, POTS, MCAS, eczema, asthma, and allergic rhinitis. While each condition brings its own challenges, they all share the need for careful management, understanding from others, and, often, advocacy on behalf of the person affected.

- Psychological Impact: Food allergy bullying can significantly affect mental health, leading to increased anxiety, fear of food-related social situations, disordered eating, a higher risk of suicide, and a lower quality of life. The added concern about potential allergic reactions makes this bullying especially important to address and validate in research.

- Potential for Physical Harm: Food allergy bullying poses a serious risk of physical harm, as even trace amounts of an allergen can trigger life-threatening reactions like anaphylaxis. In the event of food allergy bullying, it's critical to know where emergency medication is located, how to respond during a reaction, and be able to recognize the signs of an allergic reaction, which can vary significantly.

- Ignorance or Lack of Awareness: Often, food allergy bullying stems from ignorance or a lack of understanding about the seriousness of food allergies. Bullies may not realize the potential consequences of their actions, such as offering someone food containing allergens or deliberately contaminating their belongings with allergens.

- Social Isolation and Exclusion: People with food allergies often face social exclusion, which can be made worse by bullying. This affects their ability to engage in activities and feel included with peers. School counselors, therapists, and teachers must recognize this, especially for K–12 students, but it's equally relevant for adults who may experience similar challenges.

Individuals with food allergies, especially from low-income or marginalized backgrounds, face added challenges like food insecurity and a heightened risk of bullying. Systemic racism and discrimination often further complicate these issues, making their experiences even more difficult.

A 2021 study by researchers at Children's National Hospital revealed:

- 31% of children reported food allergy-related bullying when asked using a multi-item list of victimization behaviors.
- 51% of those bullied reported experiencing overt physical acts, such as allergens being waved in their face or intentionally put in their food.
- 66% reported non-physical overt victimization, including verbal teasing and threats.
- Only 12% of parents were aware their child had been bullied due to their food allergy.

Systemic racism and discrimination further exacerbate challenges for individuals with food allergies from marginalized backgrounds. While it is encouraging that there are organizations dedicated to serving marginalized and underserved, low-income communities affected by food allergies, the topic itself I hope remains a focus.

CFAAR, led by Dr. Ruchi Gupta, is notable for its research and advocacy efforts. Dr. Gupta's studies have highlighted disparities in food allergy prevalence among Black and Brown children, revealing that at the time of the study, they were 7% more likely to have food allergies compared to white children.

These findings underscore the importance of addressing equity in healthcare access and holistic care for these communities.

CFAAR not only conducts research but also collaborates with community organizations and healthcare providers to raise awareness, improve diagnosis, and advocate for policies that promote inclusivity for individuals with food allergies from all backgrounds. Their work aims to reduce disparities and equity, factoring in race and socioeconomic status, to make sure all communities have access to the care and resources needed to manage food allergies safely and effectively.

In the US "food swamps" (poor-quality food availability) and "food deserts" (no food availability) disproportionately exist where racially marginalized groups live and work. Due to this, I was particularly inspired when I discovered CFAAR and the pioneering work of Emily Brown, the former CEO and originator of the Food Equality Initiative (FEI), who worked tirelessly to provide safe foods for those in need of food assistance with allergies and celiac disease. Her efforts highlighted an overlooked gap: most food banks are not equipped to accommodate dietary needs such as life-threatening food allergies. A 2020 study by FEI revealed that out of the 60,000 food pantries nationwide, only 4 were stocked with items reserved for people in need of allergy-safe and gluten-free food.

I'm hopeful that the situation is improving, especially based on what I've observed in my local community. In Louisville, KY, I've had the privilege of volunteering with Dare to Care, a food pantry non-profit that is well-versed in food allergies and dietary restrictions. They actively uplift the food allergy community in many positive ways, and I had the pleasure of touring the kitchens to learn about how they manage food allergies.

Since the publication of the 2020 study, it seems promising that the awareness raised by COVID-19 has prompted food banks and pantries to better accommodate diverse dietary needs and rethink the ways they've been operating in the past. I truly hope this is the case, and I would love to see more recent studies and public reports reflecting these developments.

There is something people refer to as the "food allergy tax," and similar concepts like the "celiac tax" exist as well. These terms highlight a very real expense of buying safe products—foods, non-food items, lotions, and more. Having a food allergy means you can't simply take whatever is available or provided; you have to choose what is safe. For families facing food insecurity, this can quickly become overwhelming. I've seen examples of how fast costs add up: a box of cereal off the regular shelf might be affordable, but an allergen-transparent brand free of certain top allergens can be half the amount of food for double the cost. Milk is another example—while a gallon of standard milk may seem reasonable, those who can't have dairy or nut-based alternatives are often limited to rice or soy milk, which narrows options available and increases expenses. This makes the work of allergy-aware food pantries like Dare to Care all the more critical, as they provide access to safe foods for families who might otherwise go without.

It also shows why some countries, such as Italy, provide stipends for those with celiac disease to be able to buy gluten-free products. It literally costs people with celiac more to eat, and the country provides financial assistance to help even it out. Consider if this were a more common practice. Imagine how amazing it would be if a similar stipend existed for people with food allergies and other chronic dietary conditions at a more global scale, helping to offset the real costs of safe foods and giving families more security and choice.

Building Confidence and Managing Food Allergy Anxiety

Not everyone will find the same relaxation strategies effective, and that's okay. The key is to discover what works for you and your family and to intentionally schedule these practices into your routine—because life is busy. This section explores actionable ways to manage food allergy anxiety while building confidence and resilience.

Identifying and naming your fears is the first step toward managing them. For me, that often meant acknowledging thoughts like, *Will I know the symptoms of anaphylaxis when they happen?* or *Will I use my epinephrine in time?* Once these fears are named, practices such as 4-4-8 breathing (inhale for four seconds, hold for four seconds, exhale for eight seconds) or grounding exercises like the 5-4-3-2-1 method—where you notice 5 things you can see, 4 you can touch, 3 you can hear, 2 you can smell, and 1 you can taste—can help calm both body and mind. Singing, dancing, or other physical activity can also be surprisingly effective ways to reset your nervous system. Free apps like Insight Timer—a meditation app with more than 250,000 guided meditations at the time of publishing—along with its easy-to-use meditation timer, can provide additional support for calming and resetting your body and mind.

Therapeutic Approaches

Cognitive Behavioral Therapy (CBT) and Cognitive Processing Therapy (CPT) are evidence-based modalities often recommended for managing food allergy anxiety and trauma. A food-specialized therapist can also help individuals challenge avoidance behaviors, such as refraining from social events due to allergen concerns. Gradual exposure therapy under the supervision of a board-certified allergist—such as progressively eating meals closer to someone handling allergens in a controlled environment—can increase tolerance and confidence.

Building self-efficacy is another excellent tool. Practicing small steps—like speaking with chefs about ingredients, reviewing menus in advance, or carrying epinephrine confidently—can prepare you for larger challenges. These skills are part of proactive risk prevention and help individuals regain a sense of control.

Recognizing Realistic Anxiety vs. Anxiety Disorders

Food allergy anxiety is rooted in real, tangible risks, which makes it distinct from the fears often associated with anxiety disorders. Fear in this context isn't inherently negative—it can serve as a protective mechanism, keeping us alert and prepared. However, it's helpful to recognize where your anxiety lies on the spectrum—from being "careful" to going to extreme levels of being "hyper-vigilant" in a way where life begins shrinking.

Unlike anxiety disorders, which may involve irrational fears, food allergy anxiety is grounded in a valid need for caution. That said, it's important to avoid letting realistic fears spiral into catastrophic thinking, where the perception of danger outweighs the actual risks. Tools like the IDEAL framework (Identify, Define, Explore solutions, Act, Look back and reflect) can provide a practical way to evaluate concerns. By taking a step back and assessing your reactions, you can better distinguish between fears that are protective and those that may unnecessarily heighten stress.

Combating Negative Thought Patterns

Challenging unhelpful thought patterns is a powerful way to break anxiety cycles. If you find yourself stuck in a "think trap," try asking:

- "Is this thought helping me?"
- "What evidence supports or disputes this fear?"
- "What would I say to a friend feeling this way?"

Writing these reflections down in a journal or notebook you can revisit later, and practicing positive self-talk, can help reinforce healthier thought habits. For worries that linger, flipping the thought—asking, "Is this helpful? Is it even true?"—and physically discarding it (for example, tearing up a written note) can be surprisingly empowering.

Recognizing the overlap between anxiety and anaphylaxis symptoms—like a racing heart or a sense of doom—can help you tell the difference between the two. Practicing grounding exercises in calm moments, such as focusing on your senses in the present, can make them easier to use when stress is high.

Resilience, simply put, is the ability to bounce back from hard moments and is a skill that can be developed through independence and confidence-building activities. While it isn't automatic, resilience improves with practice. Tools like the Circle of Control exercise, which focuses on what you can control, such as your own actions or reactions, and gratitude journaling, where you list three things you're thankful for, can shift your perspective and reduce anxiety over time.

Remember, anxiety around food allergies doesn't just disappear. However, by focusing on what you can control and equipping yourself with practical tools, you can take meaningful steps toward a more empowered and confident life.

Closing Thoughts & Additional Context

- The Month of May: Food allergies can significantly affect mental health, leading to despondency, anxiety, fear, and feelings of exclusion, among other challenges. Addressing these emotional struggles is necessary for enhancing overall well-being. The month of May is both Food Allergy Awareness Month and Mental Health Awareness Month—a powerful reminder that these two areas are deeply connected. Living with food allergies isn't just a physical experience—it affects our emotional well-being, too. From the anxiety of eating safely to the jealousy from having to skip out on social situations, food allergies can bring both emotional highs and lows. Celebrating these awareness months together is a chance to highlight the importance of caring for our mental health just as much as our physical health. May is also Celiac Awareness Month, which reminds us of other conditions like celiac disease where strict dietary vigilance is a must. Though celiac disease is not an allergy, many of the challenges, like hidden ingredients and cross-contact, overlap. Some people in the celiac community describe it as "deadly" to make others take it seriously, but it's important to explain that reactions aren't immediately life-threatening and don't require epinephrine—and that long-term exposure to gluten can cause potentially fatal health consequences. Explaining it clearly helps others understand the risks without confusing celiac with anaphylactic food allergies.

- Fear & Anxiety: Food allergy anxiety is grounded in realistic fears and differs from unfounded fear, as it stems from legitimate risks. Managing this anxiety involves identifying personalized strategies and intentionally practicing them, such as reframing fears, grounding exercises, and building resilience. By focusing on what you can control and gradually gaining confidence, you can navigate life with food allergies more effectively and reduce the impact of anxiety on your daily experiences.

- Inadequate Labeling Issues: Our current lack of US labeling on food and non-food products makes it difficult to make informed decisions to avoid potential allergic reactions, which come with mental health consequences. Passing policies to enhance labeling practices is essential to mitigate these physical and mental health struggles.

- Financial and Healthcare Inequities: Managing food allergies can be financially burdensome for everyone involved, but especially for marginalized communities facing systemic barriers. The high costs of life-saving medications like epinephrine, doctor and hospital visits, and allergen-free foods create significant hardships for many individuals and families. These financial pressures can lead to delayed care, increased risk, and added emotional stress. If the US adopted a universal healthcare system, it could help alleviate some of this financial strain. Additionally, passing robust food allergy policies—such as mandatory allergen labeling, public education, and school-based training—would promote greater safety and awareness. Prioritizing underserved populations is essential to creating a more equitable society, where people with food allergies can thrive without stigma or avoidable danger. For those currently struggling to afford their epinephrine, the article "What if I Can't Afford My Epinephrine Medication?" by the Allergy & Asthma Network offers practical tips and potential resources to access this essential medication. This is just one example, and I even have a version on my website, invisiblyallergic.com, that outlines where to find coupons for various types of epinephrine. These articles are meant to offer guidance and support around access to medication and affordability, serving as a reminder that no one should be priced out of safety.

- Allergic Living Magazine: *Allergic Living Magazine* has become a comprehensive fully digital e-magazine resource for the food allergy community, one that many with food allergies don't know exists. They've covered almost any allergy topic you can think of, including food trauma and mental health, and have a dedicated "Food Allergy Anxiety" guide available for purchase. While the e-magazines have to be purchased, their website does have many resources, free advice, and food allergy, celiac, environmental allergies, and asthma information.

12

THE FUTURE OF ALLERGY CARE

Advancing Care, Embracing Change

Recent advancements in food allergy research and treatments are offering new hope for individuals living with these conditions. One repeat area of focus is the question of whether a mother's diet or a baby's diet has a greater influence on the development of allergic diseases.

Research suggests that a diverse, balanced diet for the mother and baby is key to promoting a healthy immune system. Studies, including work by Carina Venter, PhD, RD, emphasize that home-cooked meals are always preferable, as ultra-processed foods can negatively affect the microbiome and the gut's ability to regulate immune responses.

The "sterile" nature of store-bought foods such as applesauce, doesn't provide the same beneficial bacteria found in fresh foods, like homemade applesauce, that help to prevent allergies and diseases. Likewise, when introducing allergens, kids ideally should have the option of being able to chew and more easily spit out, rather than being prompted to swallow immediately.

For example, if you have the choice when introducing allergens, avoid the form of a smoothie or drinkable puree, to better allow for a slower, more controlled reaction if there is one. In terms of allergist advice for children, it's beneficial for our microbiome for parents to encourage diversity in their child's diet early on if possible. The Eat the Rainbow approach aligns to promote a strong immune system, because the more colorful your plate is, the more nutrients you're getting.

Additionally, recent findings show that eating a variety of plant-based foods correlates with better health outcomes and reduced disease risk. Butyrate-producing bacteria, which support immune health, are integral in this process. This isn't information shared to shame anyone doing otherwise, it's just that since there is no known cause for food allergies and no cure, this is what many of the top allergists around the globe are recommending as food for thought to help curb the development of allergic reactions.

As the medical field continues to learn more about food allergies, guidance will evolve. However, encouraging a wide variety of foods early on appears to be low-risk and will likely remain a long-term recommendation.

As children grow into adolescence, many teens begin to feel hesitant about carrying their epinephrine auto-injectors. I know I did. It's common to want to blend in, and sometimes teens downplay their allergy—especially if they haven't before experienced a severe reaction. But because anaphylaxis can happen unexpectedly, this is a critical time for open conversations between teens, their families, and their allergists. These talks can help teens better understand their allergies, while also reinforcing their strengths and autonomy. Whether you're a parent or a teen reading this, know that carrying epinephrine isn't a sign of weakness, it's a sign of being prepared and taking control of your health. It can save your life, and that's irreplaceable.

The landscape of allergy care is evolving with the use of biologics like Xolair (omalizumab). Initially developed and FDA-approved for treating moderate to severe asthma and chronic idiopathic urticaria, Xolair has also been approved as an adjunctive treatment for certain food allergies. It is an injection typically taken every 4 weeks and only works as long as the patient continues taking it.

The medicine works by binding to immunoglobulin E (IgE) antibodies, preventing them from attaching to mast cells, which therefore reduces the allergic reaction triggered by allergen exposure. While Xolair does not cure food allergies or guarantee to eliminate reactions, it can raise the threshold for allergic reactions, allowing some patients to show significant efficacy at 16-18 weeks of treatment.

However, much of the research about combining biologics with other treatments—such as those for other inflammatory diseases—has yet to be fully explored. The current gap in knowledge between rheumatologists and allergists regarding combination therapies, treatments that use multiple medications together, highlights the need for further collaboration and research on how these drugs may interact. The US medical system is so siloed, that the data doesn't exist on rheumatologists cross over with the allergy field. In general, no one medical field holistically looks at the patient, and this needs to happen in the future of patient-care, since inflammatory diseases are related.

I've heard from many allergists that overdiagnosis is a widespread issue in the food allergy community. At-home allergy tests, which people often use without consulting a board-certified allergist, are not recommended for this reason. These tests can cause unnecessary panic, leading people to eliminate foods from their diets that they don't need to avoid. As we know, food allergy tests are still not accurate enough to reliably diagnose allergies on their own.

Allergists must be cautious when diagnosing allergies, since the diagnostic process often relies heavily on exposure history paired with positive IgE levels. Oral food challenges (OFCs) are another way to determine an allergy, but they are not always implemented due to understandable concerns about triggering a reaction. Allergies are anything but cut and dry. These in-office OFCs are often considered essential to understanding the true nature of a patient's food allergies, helping to determine their tolerance levels, and guiding treatment plans—but it's also completely valid if someone doesn't feel comfortable undergoing one.

While avoidance of allergens and triggers is the only way to live safely, over-avoidance, often driven by anxiety or fear, can harm the patient's overall health and isn't as benign as one may think. For instance, unnecessarily limiting one's diet can lead to nutritional deficiencies, as individuals may avoid whole food groups that are essential for balanced nutrition. Additionally, over-avoidance can exacerbate anxiety and stress, which can negatively impact mental and physical health over time.

Another area of significant concern is the rise in adult-onset food allergies, with more individuals being diagnosed later in life. A trend that leaves adults with an abrupt social and psychological challenge, suddenly having to adjust to a completely new way of living life. FARE's state-by-state food allergy data found that the prevalence of food allergies has been increasing, with a 377% rise in anaphylactic food reactions from 2007 to 2016. This increase suggests that many individuals are developing food allergies later in life, rather than being born with them. While the exact percentages of adult-onset versus congenital food allergies are not provided in the search results, it's clear that a significant proportion of food allergies develop after childhood.

Unlike other food allergies, alpha-gal syndrome (AGS) is triggered by a tick bite, rather than developing on its own. While AGS is becoming more recognized, it remains misunderstood by many healthcare providers, including allergists. In 2023, a CDC survey uncovered a startling truth about alpha-gal syndrome (AGS): a whopping 42% of healthcare providers had never even heard of it. Among the 1,500 providers surveyed, only 5% felt "very confident" in their ability to diagnose or manage AGS, while 35% admitted they were "not too confident."

These figures are alarming—especially considering that it is estimated to affect over 450,000 Americans. It's been reported on every continent and is increasingly recognized as a global concern. Because AGS is still newly recognized, is underdiagnosed and underreported, exact numbers are difficult to determine. However, it is now ranked as the 10th most common food allergy in the US, and cases continue to rise each year.

Yet, this pervasive lack of awareness among healthcare providers not only fuels underdiagnosis but also leaves patients grappling with inadequate care and a misunderstood condition. It's a sobering reminder of the knowledge gap that still exists in the medical community about emerging allergic conditions like AGS, especially of the mental burden that comes along with it.

Patients with AGS react to mammalian-derived ingredients and these are hidden in many food and non-food products. Common culprits include gelatin, carrageenan, and certain goat and cow dairy products, which are not always clearly labeled. However, less obvious sources can also pose risks, such as certain medications or supplements, sensitivity and reactions to leather products, processed foods containing natural flavors derived from animal sources, and even cosmetics or personal care products with tallow or lanolin. This sudden lifestyle upheaval can feel isolating, overwhelming, and greatly impact social aspects, amplifying its already complex nature.

These hidden triggers make navigating AGS especially multifaceted, as they require constant vigilance beyond just reading food labels. Just like with other food allergies, AGS reactions exist on a spectrum. Some people can tolerate a certain amount of their triggers while others are highly allergic to trace amounts or are airborne reactive.

AGS is technically an allergy to "alpha-gal," a sugar molecule found in most mammals, except not humans, so our bodies can react to it when it is introduced into the human body through certain tick bites. FYI, there is no known tick bite ratio needed to develop AGS, it's been tested but still isn't known. What we do know is that this sugar exposure triggers an immune response, leading to allergic reactions from red meat and other mammal-derived products.

Regarding diagnostic advancements, blood tests for detecting alpha-gal-specific IgE antibodies are available through laboratories like LabCorp and Quest Diagnostics. These tests are instrumental in diagnosing AGS, offering an alternative to traditional skin-prick tests, which is unreliable for this allergy. For ongoing support and practical guidance, I recommend following Two Alpha Gals, who brand themselves as "your guide to living with alpha-gal syndrome" and offer a wealth of resources on their website.

From recent food allergy conferences I've attended, I learned Xolair has proven to be effective for AGS, too. As more patients put in applications for coverage, it is becoming an important part of the treatment regimen. Advances in treatments like Oral Immunotherapy (OIT) are also changing the field, although they remain mysterious and therefore controversial.

While OIT has shown promise, particularly in terms of desensitization to allergens, it is not without its risks or financial costs. The field faces major issues related to equity and access to these types of treatment, as well as concerns about the consistency and regulation of these therapies. In particular, the potential for "unregulated" OIT practices—where results are not properly tracked and patient outcomes are not reported—raises alarms. Not to mention, the methods used in OIT, TIP, and the like, aren't published for allergists to be able to understand what's being done at these clinics.

People, including allergists, hear and see these OIT and TIP-type clinics, and patients at the clinics talk about results, and it feels like magic. Without the process being transparent, it's making people skeptical. A New York allergist I heard speak at a food allergy conference has 4 patients at one of these clinics in Southern California, and all of them have signed NDAs. He's tried to get information on what they're doing at the clinic—whether it's true that their few published studies are showing 100% success rates—but they haven't disclosed their process even to him.

Due to this, it's assumed that the effectiveness of programs like OIT and TIP is often overestimated, although we don't know for sure. We need more research to assess its long-term safety and benefits, particularly in terms of reducing the need for epinephrine and emergency room visits. OIT and similar can be easily monetized while remaining unregulated and uncontrolled—issues that need to be addressed in the field.

Right now, there's no direct measuring of patients, and patient-important outcomes are vital. We need to track whether the quality of life improves, if the patient's age impacts the effectiveness, whether epi use decreases, if patients stay out of the ER, for how long they remain dosing, and how long it remains effective. Additionally, accidental deaths aren't well studied, and people often assume that OIT has more benefits than cons. But we need data to verify these assumptions.

With OIT, the formula of low and slow is typically followed abroad, as seen in a German study where no epinephrine was used and no eosinophilic esophagitis (EoE) formed. However, the treatment landscape is becoming more complex, especially in the US; with the availability of other treatments like Xolair, emphasis must be placed on patient benefits and quality. And that equity and access to OIT should be an integral part of the healthcare conversation.

The decision to pursue OIT may require years of therapy or CBT work before even deciding whether to start it. It may or may not be the right path for everyone, but we must acknowledge that OIT access varies widely and outcomes aren't guaranteed. Allergists across the US have noted a glaring discrepancy: the current published US guidelines for Oral Immunotherapy (OIT) often fail to align with many of the treatments they see being administered. In contrast, the EU has implemented stricter regulations, requiring OIT clinics to conduct thorough research and adhere to EU-specific guidelines. It's easy to see why I referred to this as a "controversy" earlier, isn't it?

As I reflect on aging with life-threatening food allergies, I wonder what accommodations will look like in 20 to 30 years. While food allergies are more widely recognized now, I can't currently imagine a nursing home free of allergens or with dedicated spaces where allergies are taken seriously. In fact, something I've only heard about, but haven't had time to explore in depth, is feeding tube regulations for people with food allergies and other allergic conditions. This highlights how many needs still remain unaddressed. As far as I can tell, there is no standardized allergen labeling for feeding tube foods.

Feeding tube formulas, also known as enteral nutrition products, are regulated by the FDA. However, these products are not subject to the same allergen labeling requirements as foods intended for oral consumption. While the FDA mandates that foods declare the presence of major food allergens on their labels, medical foods—including enteral nutrition products—are exempt from certain labeling requirements. Specifically, medical foods are exempt from the labeling requirements for health claims and nutrient content claims under the Nutrition Labeling and Education Act of 1990.

While all labeling must be accurate, truthful, and not misleading, as required by the Federal Food, Drug, and Cosmetic Act, I've learned that leaving regulations in the food allergy space as "voluntary" or vague often means additional bills must be passed later to make them mandatory, it's really the only way to ensure they actually happen.

This means that enteral nutrition products may not provide clear allergen information, which can pose real risks for individuals with food allergies who rely on them. The lack of standardized allergen labeling for feeding tube foods underscores the need for increased awareness and advocacy to ensure that people with food allergies receive safe and appropriate nutritional support, no matter their age or care setting.

It's a frightening reality—particularly in medical settings like hospitals, where I always need to remain on guard. In many situations that land you in the hospital, however, patients may be unable to advocate for themselves.

Meals in cafeteria-like settings, especially without proper allergen-protocols, can pose a significant risk, and one small oversight could be life-threatening. Worse, the medical staff would first need to inquire about an allergy, and our current labeling laws for medications and food are far from adequate. Most people aren't even aware of how insufficient these regulations are. Having someone to advocate for me during those moments has been essential. If you're over the age of 18, one helpful preventative step is to contact your local, nearby hospital and ask about adding trusted friends or family members to your medical file. This way, they can be notified and possibly involved in your care if you end up in the hospital unexpectedly.

Perhaps accommodating senior facilities already exists on a small scale, like nut-free college campuses are beginning to, so they may become more common in the future. Only time will tell. For now, many care centers and medical facilities still face challenges in accommodating food allergies. In these situations, the food allergy adult often finds themselves in the position of acting as the expert, navigating the complexities of their condition, even while they are the patient. Navigating the emotional back-and-forth of being both the expert on the diagnosis and the patient in need of care can be exhausting.

Finally, research into the structural impacts of allergies on the brain is a growing area of interest. Studies on conditions like inflammatory bowel disease (IBD) and celiac disease have started to explore the gut-brain axis, which has found structural changes in the brain due to these conditions. There is still limited data on how food allergies might affect brain function over time, but if our brains are changing due to these conditions, it's natural to wonder what other aspects of our mind-body connection could be impacted. Understanding the link between food allergies and mental health—especially the anxiety and depression that often accompany conditions like alpha-gal syndrome (AGS) and celiac disease—is crucial for developing comprehensive care plans.

I've been inspired by the increasing conversation around food allergies in the mainstream and the innovation happening in this space. I hope that this progress continues, particularly with a focus on equity in access. Sadly, those who need medical care the most are often the ones unable to receive it in the US due to financial barriers. I'm inspired by companies like Kitt Medical, based in the UK, which provides life-saving epinephrine in a way similar to how defibrillators and fire extinguishers are available. While there are some efforts in the US to pass bills for epinephrine in public spaces like schools, there's still a significant gap in healthcare access for those who need it.

As I close this final chapter, I reflect on the power of stories to inspire change. Food allergies are not just a medical condition; they are a lens through which we can view broader issues of equity, accessibility, and innovation. The journey to improve food and non-food labeling laws, address disparities in healthcare, and raise awareness about the life-altering impacts of food allergies is far from over. Yet, every small victory—every conversation that sparks understanding, every policy that prioritizes safety, and every advocate who takes a stand—builds a foundation for a more inclusive and equitable future. I hope that this book leaves readers with not just awareness, but also a sense of urgency to be part of the solution. Together, we can create a world where life-threatening food allergies are met with the compassion, knowledge, and systemic support they deserve.

Access to allergy specialists, and even just basic healthcare, remains a significant barrier, with an estimated one allergist per 65,000 people in the US. It's been pointed out that allergists have the unique opportunity to address the body holistically with multidisciplinary approaches, as they often address the whole person—skin, gut, and respiratory issues in tandem.

The US continues to lag behind the EU in incorporating patient voices into research, healthcare policy, and allergy management guidelines—even in areas as basic as access to fresh, affordable produce. But the food allergy field is still so new that no one country has completely figured it out. Some countries do offer food allergy or celiac stipends to help offset the cost of allergen-safe foods and provide additional healthcare benefits for those diagnosed. In certain places, it's also common practice for doctors to prescribe a probiotic alongside an antibiotic—an approach that reflects an awareness of the gut's role in overall health, including immunity and allergic reactivity. Still, be skeptical of anyone marketing supplements as a "cure" for food allergies. We're simply not there yet, and for now, that's not the reality.

We're just beginning to understand how gut health, microbiome diversity, and early exposures might shape allergic outcomes. It feels like we're on the precipice of major breakthroughs, but also in the midst of figuring it all out in real time. Globally, we're all tackling this together. Advocating for increased funding to organizations doing the work you want to see more of is crucial. These efforts can help address disparities and improve outcomes for future generations.

We can now so clearly see how food allergies impact identity and community deeply. Within the allergy community, fatalities are in many ways felt as heavy familial losses, as we know so easily how this could happen to any of us. If you grew up with a food allergy, these conditions shape self-perception early on, especially during formative years when children wrestle with questions like, "Who am I with this condition?" At a recent food allergy conference I attended, the point was made that no one labels a kid as "cancer kid" or "lupus kid," but being noted as the "food allergy kid" is done effortlessly and often defines children in a uniquely isolating way, tethered to constant vigilance, worriedness, and a label of over-caution.

It's equally important to combat common societal misconceptions—dismissive comments like "everyone has allergies nowadays" or "I have food allergies, but I just eat my allergens anyway" undermine the seriousness of IgE-mediated allergies and highlight the need for additional food allergy education.

This labeling even happens with adults; heck, I've even done it to myself! If someone has accommodated my allergy and I later meet them in person for the first time, I've caught myself introducing myself as *I'm the one with the peanut allergy you emailed with,* emphasizing it in a way I wouldn't for other conditions. For adults with adult onset food allergies, the transition from living a life without any fear of food to having to develop and learn all these habits, tips, tricks, and ingredient labeling laws is a monumental transition that doesn't get enough attention.

The reality is that food allergies represent a profound loss of control, and so regaining empowerment where we can in life is often essential for grounding ourselves. Practices like oral food challenges or testing for related allergens can help restore food confidence and lead to greater dietary diversity. However, trauma often accompanies these conditions—particularly after anaphylaxis—but even just seeing someone go into anaphylaxis can be traumatic. For food-allergic individuals and their circles, this can so easily lead to anxiety and panic, and it is where many find themselves, understandably living in a certain level of life-limiting fear. Avoidance of foods becomes common but can evolve into excessive avoidance of full categories of food, underscoring the need to challenge allergy anxiety in a way that works with the person's quality of life.

Food allergy parents can play a key role in managing the psychological impacts of an allergy, too. By asking open-ended questions like, "How are you feeling?" or "Are you scared?" they can support their child without projecting their fears onto them. Encouragement to embrace life, despite food trauma, is vital. As I often remind myself: food allergies are serious, but you still get to live your life. It may look different than some other's lives, but that's okay, what a boring world it would be if we were all the same.

Practical strategies can help mitigate emotional burdens within the allergy and food allergy disability community. Affirmations like, "I know how to handle a reaction," paired with calming techniques such as deep breathing, can help lessen self-blame and fearfulness.

Recognizing the evolving nature of medical knowledge— *What I know today may be completely different a week from now*—is grounding, especially in a field defined by uncertainty. Managing allergies requires bridging both art and science, and tools like AI. While it scares me in many aspects, AI may one day revolutionize patient care. While I'm not fully counting on it, AI's potential to analyze medical data in unprecedented ways has opened my mind to possibilities I've never imagined. I hope companies can harness this technology responsibly and sustainably for the long-term health of our planet.

The online world is full of complexities: misinformation, algorithms steering us toward polarized content, and the enticing allure of technology. Navigating it all can feel overwhelming. Built to be addictive, with features like infinite scrolling, these platforms make me find myself grappling with a new reality. The rapid evolution of AI blurs the lines of authenticity, leaving me to question what is real and what isn't—prompting me to question what I'm seeing and to read more deeply than I ever did a decade ago. In this landscape, cultivating the practice of slowing down has become necessary for my mental health.

I often feel like I'm racing through life at a frenetic pace, but for what purpose? As I draw this final chapter of my memoir to a close, I hold tightly to the belief that all voices matter and that each person holds the same high value. No one is above another; each person is someone else's world.

Change never happens at the pace we think it should. It happens over years of people joining together, strategizing, sharing, and pulling all the levers they possibly can. Gradually, excruciatingly slowly, things start to happen, and then suddenly, seemingly out of the blue, something will tip.

—Judy Heumann

If you give people the spark of possibilities, that spark becomes a big flame of hope.

—José Andrés

A Final Word

As the field of allergy research—especially regarding food allergies—advances at a remarkable pace, fueled by organizations like Food Allergy Science Initiative (FASI) and the National Institute of Allergy and Infectious Diseases (NIAID), I can envision a future where desensitization to allergens becomes the norm. It's an outlook I never would have imagined possible during those harrowing moments of anaphylaxis on the allergist's table, feeling so isolated in my quest to find safe foods just 11 years ago.

If you had told me a year ago that my purse would contain two Neffy nasal-spray, needle-free epinephrine medications, I wouldn't have known how to react. To be honest, I'm still coming to terms with it. Out of hesitancy to trust a new product, lately I've been carrying both the Neffy nasal spray epinephrine and my traditional auto-injectors—embracing this new reality that seems almost surreal. The thought of it brings happy tears to my eyes, as the fears of my childhood flood back to the forefront of my mind. I can still recall my doctor explaining, in a positive tone, that I should feel relieved my auto-injector could penetrate three layers of ski gear.

As I looked down at my petite frame, adorned in shorts and a tank top, devoid of extra skin and never having skied, I was gripped by anxiety at her comment. My throat tightened, my stomach dropped, and I felt my body temperature plummet a few degrees. "Was there a version designed for wearing regular clothes, rather than thick layers?" I asked. "No, no, it's a good thing; you can use it even if you have a lot of layers," she replied. Still, that did little to reassure me.

I couldn't shake the unsettling, graphic image of the needle hitting my bone or plunging too deep and emerging on the other side of my thigh. I knew this likely wouldn't be my reality, but as I stared down at my exposed legs, dread washed over me. I carried this comment with me through high school and into adulthood, frequently glancing down at my jeans or leggings and worrying about whether I'd need to use my epinephrine injector, feeling vulnerable without having on thick winter gear.

I remember a few years later, reading over the epinephrine pamphlet and learning that the injector would work for me at just 80 pounds—barely surpassing the 66-pound child limit—yet was also suitable for a 300-pound adult. The fear I experienced as a child and young adult, transitioning from the EpiPen Jr. with its smaller dose to the larger auto-injector, was overwhelming. I remember asking my doctors to stay on the EpiPen Jr. dosage, feeling so small and un-adult-like in my body. They reassured me repeatedly that the regular dose was perfectly fine, but I panicked at the thought of having to use the device.

Now, heading into 2026, well into my thirties and equipped with my skill set of navigating the world with a peanut allergy and the wisdom that comes with it, I find myself excited for a safe cure—if one were to develop—but not counting on one. My primary focus remains on promoting societal acceptance and creating meaningful accommodations for all individuals, regardless of their unique health challenges.

By recognizing how food allergies touch the lives of many, we can cultivate a society that ensures that no one feels isolated by their circumstances. While no one asks to be different, we must embrace our individuality and see the beauty in our diverse experiences.

As you reflect on the information in this book, I invite you to join the movement for greater awareness and understanding of food allergies. Your voice and support can help amplify the message of safety and acceptance. Sharing your personal experiences—whether as someone with food allergies or as a supporter of those who live with them—can create a powerful narrative.

Let us continue to cultivate resilience, share our truths, and practice solidarity because together, we can create a future where compassion paves the way for everyone to thrive and live fearlessly. The road ahead may be winding and long, but with unity and a persistent unwavering spirit, we will forge a path toward a world where food allergies are met with respect.

Key Points & Reflections

- Advancements In Food Allergy Treatment: The field of food allergy treatment rapidly advancing, with multiple forms of management options and promising technologies like sublingual versions of epinephrine on the horizon. These developments offer hope for greater empowerment, treatment, and improved safety for those living with food allergies, especially because sublingual forms could be more accessible for people who struggle with traditional injection methods. Historically, epinephrine (adrenaline) was only administered in hospitals via syringes and ampules (sealed glass capsules containing a liquid). The introduction of self-carry epinephrine auto-injectors revolutionized emergency care, making life-saving treatment more readily available and easy to use without medical training. However, these injectors—such as EpiPen or newer options like Neffy nasal spray—still require a certain level of grip strength, dexterity, and coordination. This can be a significant barrier for people with disabilities, arthritis, or other conditions that affect hand function. Sublingual forms of epinephrine offer a much easier and more accessible alternative for these individuals. In addition, FDA-approved biologics like Xolair offer hope for reducing severe allergic reactions by targeting the immune response. These advances represent meaningful progress in food allergy management, especially for individuals who have struggled to find effective solutions for life-threatening reactions. As of this writing, many allergists in the US have shared that they look to the European Academy of Allergy and Clinical Immunology (EAACI)'s 2024 guidelines for IgE-mediated food allergy as a key international resource to help create more uniform standards for allergy treatment worldwide. I plan to continue checking the EAACI's guidelines each year to stay informed about their recommended best practices.

- A Diverse Diet Is Key: As much as we can, eating more fresh, homemade meals and having less processed foods is best for fostering a diverse and healthy microbiome. The emphasis on plant-based foods and avoiding overly processed options is gaining traction as part of a comprehensive approach to immune health and disease prevention, even when it comes to developing food allergies.

- Importance of Education and Combating Misconceptions: Dismissive societal comments trivialize life-threatening allergies and highlight the need for better allergy education. Both children and adults face unique challenges, such as transitioning to life with adult-onset allergies or managing stigma and fear.

- The Role of Caregivers and Community Support: Parents and caregivers can support children by asking open-ended questions, encouraging self-expression, and avoiding projecting their own fears. Affirmations and grounding techniques can help individuals regain confidence and manage anxiety around allergens. The #1 resource I suggest for any parent or caregiver new to navigating food allergies with a child is Free to Feed, which offers practical guidance, expert advice, and support to help families feel confident and empowered.

- Cultivating Resilience and Solidarity: Food allergies reveal the importance of compassion and acceptance in creating a society where no one feels isolated. Sharing personal experiences and raising awareness can build understanding and pave the way for lasting societal change.

- A Call to Action: Amplifying voices within the food allergy community and promoting safety and inclusion are critical steps toward creating a more equitable future. Advocacy and solidarity can help shape a world where food allergies are respected and managed with empathy and care.

Acknowledgments

I am deeply thankful to everyone who supported me in this creative venture. To my partner, Paul, thank you for believing in me and encouraging me to launch *Invisibly Allergic* to begin with. Your unwavering faith in my abilities gave me the guts to embark on this writing journey and share my voice with the world. Thank you for always being in my corner and for helping make all my dreams come true—this book and so many others.

I am also profoundly grateful to my close friends and family for your invaluable feedback and constant encouragement throughout the writing process. Your unwavering support of my passion project, *Invisibly Allergic*, has meant the world to me. To the readers and supporters of my blog and social media platforms, your engagement and enthusiasm have fueled my passion for advocacy in countless ways.

Finally, a heartfelt thank you to the experts, healthcare professionals, and organizations dedicated to food allergy research and education, as well as the policymakers and advocates championing inclusive, open-minded initiatives. Your efforts are paving the way for meaningful change—not only within the food allergy community, but far beyond it—and your dedication continues to improve lives every day.

With deepest appreciation,
Zoë Katherine Slaughter

www.ingramcontent.com/pod-product-compliance
Lightning Source LLC
LaVergne TN
LVHW010309070526
838199LV00065B/5493